AF344292

Broken Wing

You can't quit. Not ever.

A true story of courage and inspiration.

Shawn Withers

with Sylvia Sims

Belfast, Maine US

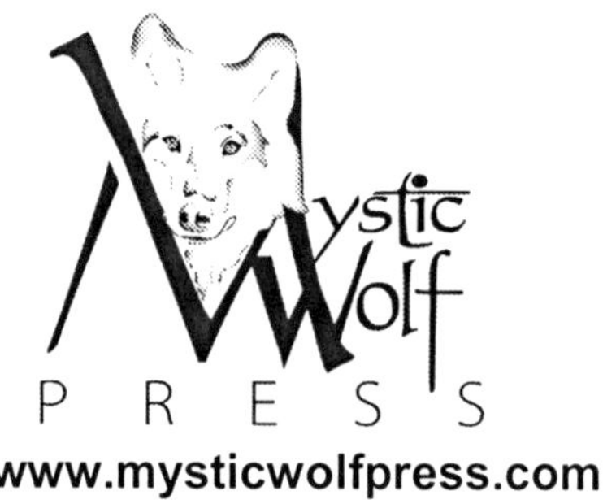

www.mysticwolfpress.com

ISBN 978-0-9790400-4-7
LCCN

Published by Mystic Wolf Press, Inc.

Printed in the United States of America.

The mind must command the limbs
and convert itself into a force that controls the
body
even if part of the body refuses to obey.

Those who let themselves go in these
circumstances
quickly fall prey to death.

There is no way out
other than remaining master of one's body
down to the last muscle.

From *In the Land of White Death*
Valerian Albanov

Foreword

I met Shawn at a seminar in Maine with James Bouchard at his school Northern Chi. Shawn came up to me and introduced himself, we talked, and became friends. Right away, I was impressed with his positive attitude and wonderful personality. Over the years, he has constantly shown his desire to help others, never complains about anything, and is always looking for the "good" in life. Shawn has been one of my students since the time we met. He went through the requirements to become a Canemaster, passed with flying colors, and has adapted to teaching others despite his partial paralysis. Shawn has a "never give up" attitude, as well as doing his best to help others where ever he goes. If the world had more people like Shawn, it would be a much better place! I feel proud and privileged that he is one of my Canemasters, and a good friend!

GrandMaster Mark Shuey, Sr., Owner of Cane Masters and Founder CMIA

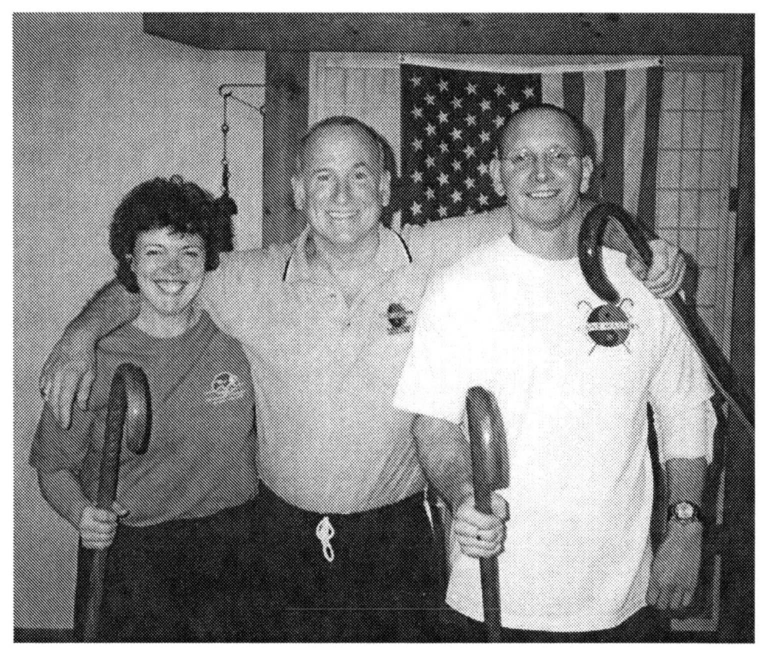

Andrea and Shawn with Grandmaster Mark Shuey, Sr.

Acknowledgements

I'd like to thank my wife, Andrea, for her endless support in my pursuit of martial arts and in the process of writing this book. Without her, I would never have accomplished these things.

I would also like to thank all my family and friends being there when I needed them most.

Contents

Part I .... **xv**

July 22, 1982 1

The Hospital 5

R4 13

Rehab 18

Home 27

Kathi's Story 31

Part II **40**

Recovery and Discovery................................... 41

Marriage and College 51

Martial Arts 59

Moving Up 69

Christopher Keith... 79

Cardiac Trouble 86

The Waiting Room.. 103

Black Belt 111

Part III **116**

Like Water...117

Student and Teacher Stories 129

Student Stories 129

Volunteer Teachers 147

Broken Wing Kenpo 151

Afterword 156

Introduction

When you meet Shawn Withers in his Dojo wearing his colorful *gi* and the black belt with the two red stripes that indicate his rank as a second degree black belt in Kenpo Karate, you don't notice anything unusual about him at first. Demonstrating a combination with blocks, strikes and kicks with lightning speed, he dances across the carpeted floor with grace and agility. As he explains the moves to his students, his face lights up with enthusiasm and his gray-blue eyes sparkle behind his glasses as he emphasizes a point. Then you observe that the left side of his face is not quite so mobile as the right, he walks with a hitch and he makes all his strikes and blocks with his well-muscled right arm while his thinner left arm curls in front by his belt.

Shawn suffered a massive, left-sided stroke at the age of twenty. He could have taken disability payments and done absolutely nothing for the rest of his life, but one night when he was lying in his hospital bed, unaware that his left side was totally flaccid, he tried to get out and walk. He fell, grabbing the bedside table and spilling a full urinal over himself. As he was lying helplessly on the floor, soaked with urine, he vowed that he was going to fight this illness; to overcome the paralysis and get on with his life. Slowly, painfully, he dragged himself to a sitting position with his right hand, pulled himself up on his good leg and fell into bed.

This is his story of how he strove to rise above his disability and succeeded, over and above his—or anybody else's—expectations. Having achieved an amazing success in an incredibly demanding art associated only with those who are physically gifted and supremely agile, he turned around and started to teach to others what he had adapted superbly to his own disabilities—not only to those who had suffered strokes as he had, but to adults and children with MS, the blind, the mentally challenged, the arthritic, the para- and quadriplegic. He has grown from a terrified, half-paralyzed, brain-damaged twenty-year-old without prospects or qualifications for a future, into a successful businessman and renowned martial artist who is evolving a new form of martial arts: Broken Wing Kenpo, a system relevant to both those with and without physical disabilities.

Others also relate their own stories about Shawn in these pages: his family, his doctors, nurses, therapists, masters of martial arts, fellow students and volunteer instructors. But above all, this is his story . . . and the stories of those whom he has helped immeasurably.

Sylvia Sims

Part l

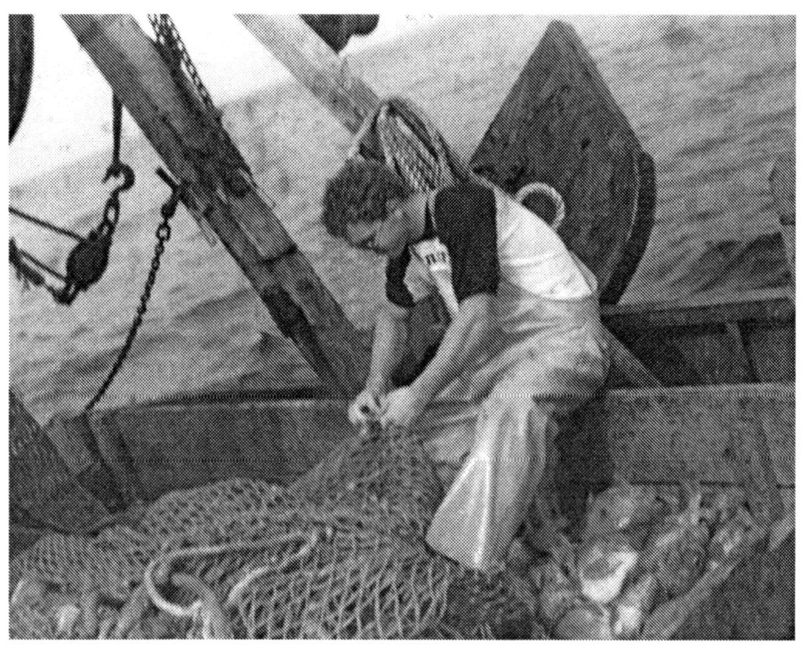

On my father's boat

1

July 22, 1982

It's midsummer: a beautiful, sunny, warm day, just a little after lunch. I'm at Fort Williams with my good friends Dave and Todd, just hanging out shootin' the shit, talking about our plans for the future; not the far-off future as we are young and only interested in the immediate, but just our plans for the fall—

Suddenly a sharp pain and severe pressure grips the front of my head; feels like a splitting mall driving into my skull. We get in the car and head for Dave's house. I'm puzzling over what could be causing this headache. Hangover? No, we hadn't gone out the night before. Migraine? Don't know—never had one. Haven't really done anything to cause this. Must be just a really bad headache but it's getting worse. I'll take care of it with some aspirin.

At Dave's house I manage to get out of the car but have to lean against it. I slip, but Todd catches me to prevent the car from being scratched. Dizzy. No balance. Feel like I'm losing part of my body, which is fighting against the loss as if I have just run 100 miles and am extremely fatigued. Someone says, "Maybe sunstroke?" Go through the garage to the kitchen to get water. Dave tells me I am dragging my foot but it doesn't feel that way to me.

I set the glass down and bang it around. I'm feeling fuzzy. Dave suggests I sit down but my balance and perception are off and I miss the chair and knock it into the other chairs and then push the table into the wall and land on the floor. This terrifies me. I can see my foot not moving and I panic. I tell my friends to leave me alone, that I'm all right, but they help me up and take me into the garage, where they put me down on the floor because it is cool. I have what I find out later is a grand mal seizure. Violent shaking of my body. Good and evil fighting it out within me. Suddenly . . . complete absence of activity. My mind is calm. My body is still and my left side is flaccid.

I hear someone telling Dave to get his mother. She's asking me if I'm okay and I tell her I don't know.

I think she's calling the ambulance. There are faces looking down at me. I can hear people talking at me but I can't communicate very well. I think my mind is clear. I can see all that is happening, but I can't make any connections. After a while I fade.

The ambulance people come and it's like waking up from a bad dream. There are people all over me and it's a rush! It's a huge commotion and it is happening right over me! I think they are taking my vitals and putting ECG leads on my body. They are slugging me in the face to get me to respond. They might be little taps but I'm not thinking clearly. They're trying to keep me awake and it is irritating me no end. They're putting oxygen on me and I'm trying to pull it off. They're jabbing me with needles and asking me about taking drugs and asking and asking all sorts of questions, overloading my mind and making me very irritable.

One calm voice is telling me I will be all right. Someone who works on the ambulance who I think I've known a long time. I hear her voice amid this sea of confusion.

They put me on a stretcher and load me into the ambulance. I hear the sirens and feel the bumpy ride. I'm trying to regroup; still feeling panic but my reasoning skills are returning. My inner voice is telling me to slow down and try to figure out what is happening. I hear the familiar sound of the grate in the middle of the Million-Dollar Bridge from South Portland and know I'm headed into Portland and it orients me a little.

In the ER at Maine Medical Center I am transferred from the stretcher to the gurney in the trauma room. More needles. That agitates me again. People are putting cold cloths on my face and trying to keep me awake. A slightly-built young doctor is asking me to move my arms and legs. He's asking me if I can feel his touch on them. Things are getting fuzzy and I am fading out again. My family is starting to gather in the ER. I keep hearing my brother Jeff's voice telling me to put my arm back on the gurney and he keeps putting it up beside me but it flops over again. I hear the panic in my mother's voice. I hear my friends' voices, too.

By the time I'm transferred to a room in the hospital I'm exhausted and don't remember any more until I wake up and feel sheer panic. I think the sheets are tucked in too tightly—perhaps I am restrained. I can't move and I freak out. My parents are there and they keep telling me to rest. I fade in and out.

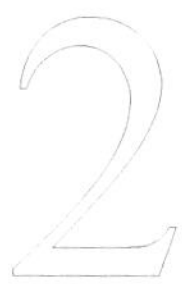

The Hospital

A journey of a thousand miles
must begin with a single step.

Lao-tzu,
from The Way of Lao-tzu

I was unaware of it for several days, but I later found out I had suffered an occluded middle cerebral artery with left hemiplegia; in layman's terms, a stroke with left-sided paralysis. I was admitted to Maine Medical Center's P2A floor from the ER early the next morning.

John Kelly Sullivan, MD—the slight young doctor—remembers that day:

I first saw Shawn in July '82 in the ER at MMC. He had suffered a massive stroke at the age of twenty.

Born with an abnormal congenital cardiac condition, his aortic semilunar valve located at the base of the ascending aorta had only two instead of the usual three half-moon-shaped leaves, or flaps, that close when the left ventricle relaxes to prevent the back flow of blood from the aorta into the left ventricle. This is usually no problem until later in life, but Shawn's had already suffered some wear that probably caused some fibrous material to form on a stalk. Eventually it broke off and flowed through his arterial system until it blocked an artery in the right side of his brain to cause a massive stroke affecting his left side. Devastating at any age but even more so at the age of twenty.

In 1982 I had only been practicing for two years and was still very young and slight in appearance. I remember having to face Shawn's father and brother who were two huge lobster-men (they were actually fishermen) and feeling very intimidated physically as I had to tell them that Shawn had had a massive stroke and would never recover the abilities he had before the stroke.

There were two issues of great concern that I had to discuss with them during Shawn's hospitalization: his need for lifetime anticoagulation and his wild character. He had a reputation for working and playing hard, drinking and 'partying'—as is common with 20-year-old males—and taking risks with his physical activities. On anticoagulants to prevent further clots forming, he was at risk for bleeding with any injury, and alcohol worsened the risk. Both Richard Anderson, his cardiologist at that time, and I were worried.

—

For several days, I was confused and very angry. Between constant testing and doctors' examinations, combined with the left-sided paralysis, I had no idea of what had happened or what was going to happen to me—I was scared. All I wanted was to go home and rest. Worse, my family had little familiarity with stroke and the doctors could not come up with a satisfactory explanation as to how it happened.

My father says:

His mother and I, as well as the rest of the family, were so scared and worried. Jeanette thought he had blood poisoning, and I didn't know what to think. It was explained to us what had happened. Shawn had had a stroke. He couldn't stand. He couldn't do anything that he had done before. His brain was damaged and so was the left half of his body. He wasn't expected to get much better and we were advised to apply for Social Security and SSDI for him. We didn't understand—old people had strokes, not a young hellion like Shawn.

—

I think I was on a regular floor for about a week before going to a rehabilitation unit. I was totally unaware of the passing of time because I was so disoriented and confused. Day or night, the perception of time—they all blurred together. At first I was told to rest and do nothing. The more they wanted me to rest, the more restless I became and—because they wanted me to rest—my mother made sure I didn't get a lot of company. I also needed rest so that the swelling in my brain would go down. When someone did visit, it left me drained and totally exhausted but I kept thinking that, if I could get home, I would get better. Nurses and doctors ask a lot of short-term memory questions but I had no short-term memory. I recognized my family but couldn't remember who visited and when. The medical records state: "only slightly confused." I admit that I must have had some acting abilities as I couldn't remember what I had eaten ten minutes before. It seemed as if there was an endless parade of physicians coming in to check me out.

"What day is this?"

"What did you have for your last meal?"

"Who is the President of the United States?"

I told them I didn't care. The sad truth was that I did not know and I was trying to cover up. Everyone kept telling me that I had a stroke. What did I know about stroke? I was way too young to have one of those. It was an old person's disease!

Nights were excruciatingly long. I could never get comfortable and kept turning over on my left arm. With the lack of sensation in my arm it was difficult to keep track of it: the doctors called it left-sided neglect. I must have been close to the nurse's station as it was quite noisy at night. Sometimes one of the nurses would give me a back-rub to relax me so I could sleep. There were no visitors at night and I was trapped in this foreign place. TV resembled static and made absolutely no sense to me.

My cousin Michael had cancer and happened to be in the hospital at that same time to receive chemotherapy treatments. He would visit me and we would laugh together as here we both were, trapped in the same place! Men did not cry together then—at least, not in our family. We were both so young to have such awful stuff happen to us; he was only three years older than me.

I remember that I had to wear a restraining (Posey) belt to keep me from falling out of bed as my left side didn't seem to exist any more. When reminded that I did have a left arm and leg, I didn't want to be aware of them and refused to look at either. I was always having blood drawn and being taken for tests. It was quite an effort to get me into a wheelchair for these tests because I always felt that I could do more than I really could, and every time I was moved around I thought they were changing my room. That led to more confusion. It was especially discomforting when I was taken for an angiography. I had no idea what was going on and having needle sticks in my groin, then feeling the dye go in with an extremely warm feeling as if I was wetting myself, was confusing as well as embarrassing. I was nearing my breaking point with this incessant testing. Always being tested; always being asked what I ate, how much I urinated or if I had moved my bowels. It was degrading. To say I was angry would be far too mild.

I found that I needed other people's assistance to do absolutely everything; very demoralizing as I had never needed anyone's help before. I had to have help just to change my underwear. This was intensely personal stuff to a twenty-year-old and it was very humiliating to be helped to the bathroom or assisted in the shower by a nurse.

It seemed to me that I should be able to do anything, but in reality I couldn't. For example, I reached out to grab something, missed, and fell out of my chair. It was yet another indication to me that I was not in control, causing more doubts, frustration and anger at myself and the people around me. Why *me*? I was a good person. I worked hard and played hard — a typical twenty-year-old without responsibilities. True, I had been born prematurely with a heart defect that did restrict some physical activities in school, but I was able to lift weights and was considered strong and fit — fit enough to go commercial fishing with my father during the winter and spring and in the summer lobstering with my cousin Gary. I worked long days and nights and was away from home for days at a time. When I came home flush with dollars I would go out with friends to bars to have fun or there was always a party going on somewhere. I had known that eventually I would want to do more with my life and regarded this playtime as temporary; still, I wanted to end it on my terms.

Vaguely I can remember my mother helping me with my food. I think she would get it ready for me, opening the packages and setting them up on the bedside table. It was always a treat when my family brought in food from McDonald's or Burger King. I never had a problem with chewing and with eating anything in front of me, as I knew that I had to eat to keep up my strength. The left side of my face was numb (and still is) and it took me several tries to clean it because my coordination was off, so family and friends got in the habit of signaling when I had some food on the left side of my face.

I don't remember having a roommate in those first days, but later there was an older gentleman who took me under his wing. He called the nurse when I couldn't find the call bell and also made sure I got what I needed, but the days of resting—quietly or not—in my bed were coming to an end. My world which had been shrunk to this tiny hospital room was about to expand.

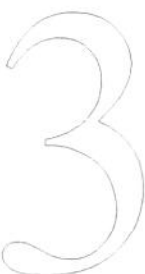

R4

> Heroism . . . is endurance for one moment more.
>
> *George Kenman,*
> *from a Letter to Henry Munro Rogers*

On August 2nd, I was moved to a rehabilitation floor—Richard's Wing 4—for therapy. I was excited but apprehensive, as I wasn't quite sure what was going to happen there or what I would be doing. I couldn't understand why I was still in the hospital. Why couldn't I go home and exercise to get better? I had always worked out and kept in great shape, and I didn't believe this situation was that much different. I thought I was going to R4 for a good workout; all I needed were some weights to start building my strength back.

I was in for a surprise.

An escort parked my wheelchair in front of the nurse's station on R4, right next to the wheelchair of another young man. It was my first close contact with another patient other than my roommate on P2A. This young man's hair was shaved off half his head. There was a scar completely circling the shaven area and some sort of a pressure gauge was stuck in the top of his head. He was rambling, making no sense to me. I had never seen anything like this. It resembled a crazy world in a movie and my adrenaline kicked in: I was going to have to be strong to survive this. Nothing the future would hold would ever bother me like this did. I could only compare it to a first day in prison—and I hadn't done anything wrong! It was way out of my limited experience with medicine and hospitals (apart from my hospitalizations for my cardiac and hernia problems when I was an infant of which I had no memory) and it was terrifying to a formerly healthy person. Eventually I became accustomed to the sights and sounds of R4; the nurses were all great-looking and very good to me, but my first impression never went away.

Georgann Dickey, RN (one of the good-looking nurses) remembers me well. She was a very young nurse at the time of my CVA, working on R4 and one of my caregivers.

> *Shawn was quiet; brooding at first, but he had a sense of humor and he had determination. He was always respectful, polite and overall, patient for a teenager. I did sense anger, but he seemed to channel this to therapy. I remember when he had his first shower since his admission. He said it was like heaven! Once he got into rehab, he started to have fun with the staff and with the other patients.*

Because I had fallen out of a chair and was not good at sitting still for long periods of time, I always needed a Posey belt to keep me in bed. Unhappy about that, I decided to fix it. I had a plan to leave this nightmare from hell! Waiting until dinner was brought, I took the knife and hid it in my pillow. That night, I cut the belt. I had observed how the side-rail was lowered by pressing the button, then I got my right leg over the side of the bed and dragged my left side over to reach for the table. It had never occurred to me that the table was on wheels. It moved. I slipped and fell to the floor. As I fell, a full urine jug that was on the table spilled all over me. I was now sitting on the floor, soaked in piss—angry and *feeling* pissed!— looking around to see if I had woken anyone up. I hadn't. My roommate was still snoring and the chatter from the nurse's station hadn't stopped. I tried to get up, but couldn't. This was the moment when I finally realized just how bad off I was.

I dragged my body to the bedside, groped above me and clamped my right arm on the rail, hoisted my body up and managed to crawl back into bed. I took off the wet johnny and never said a word to anyone, but I vowed right then and there I was going to get better and get out of here.

On August 12, I was told that someone was going to come and talk to me. I was not sure who he was, what he would do or could do for me, and I felt fine but my mother and the staff wanted me to speak to this person. Later on that day a man came to visit and he continued to do so every afternoon for many days.

It was some time before it dawned on me that he was a shrink, but he assured me that everything we spoke about would be confidential. My doctors and my parents were concerned how my 'having fun and partying' habits would affect my need for ongoing anticoagulant therapy. They also wanted me to try to get some of the anger out of my system. This shrink didn't attempt to preach to me; he just laid out the information, told me that it was my choice to take it or leave it and in doing so, he gave me back some of the control over myself that I had sorely missed during my stay in the hospital.

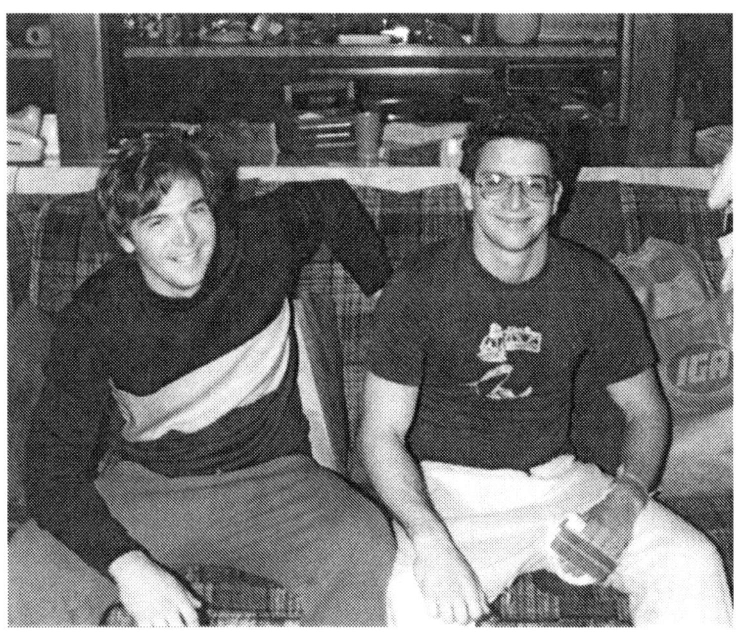

After the stroke, with my brother Jeff Withers

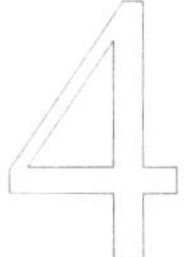

Rehab

You gain strength, courage and confidence
by every experience
in which you stop to look fear in the face.

Eleanor Roosevelt,
from You Learn by Living

I worked from the mat every day, finding to my surprise that something as simple as sitting up was now so difficult. Now I had to learn to crawl just like a baby! I kept crashing onto my left side.

Balancing, sitting—amazing how the brain tricks you into thinking you are doing so much better than you are. After what seemed to be 4,000 tries in a million hours I could finally sit up, and it was time to get off the mat.

Now I had to face the parallel bars with a mirror front of me to show me my posture. I was not a pretty sight. Physically I had become extremely frail—skin and bones with no muscle tone. I lasted less than a minute in an upright position in the first attempt without the leg brace. I felt as if I would never get this balancing act down, especially on the left side.

Slowly I started to stand more or less straight, after days and days of doing the same thing over and over again—four little steps. Four steps up and four down; not easy to do balancing and moving a leg that didn't want to work. Add to that a left arm that also didn't want to move, which made it even harder. Every time the therapists asked me to perform a particular movement I would say, "No problem." They must have been laughing inside, as I had no idea of how hard it was going to be, but I had the will and I got stronger every day.

The Physical Therapy room seemed to grow smaller and smaller after the frustration of doing the same thing over and over—then over and over again. With a lot of patience it finally started to work, a little at a time, though "baby steps" doesn't even describe it. But I *had* to keep going in order to reach the goals I had set for myself, which were to be able to move and walk as well as I had before the stroke.

Crutches. I expected them to be humiliating but at least they enabled me to stand by myself. I was so tired of the wheelchair, which was difficult to steer with one working arm. The crutches looked good. At first a few steps . . . then halfway down the hall . . . then crash! I gave everything I had every day to therapy because I knew if I worked hard I was on the way to independence.

After I became competent with the crutches, then came the cane; a little less supportive than the crutches, but I was now stronger and quicker. I had freedom back at last! With a cane I could go anywhere so I walked and walked.

Recreational Therapy, however, was disappointing. There were Ping-Pong and playing cards, but I needed help as I could hold only a few cards in one hand. The other patients were a diverse group of people with problems that ranged from brain injury to para- and quadriplegia. I had never been around people who had such physical problems before and to me this was a very scary place, so I just kept to myself in the first few weeks. All I intended to do was my job of recovery and then go home. The therapists wanted me to go to group sessions, but I didn't want to socialize with anyone as I felt I was there only to work on my physical abilities. The other patients were far worse off than I was. Sometimes denial is good as it is our way of protecting ourselves from things that are too painful to cope with at the time. I didn't realize until later that I was in the same boat that all the other patients were; that I had to break down the walls I had put up to protect myself from pain and face my demons in order to get better.

A gorgeous blonde recreational therapist was persistent and patient with me, chipping away at my walls but letting me keep my pride. She finally persuaded me to go to a magic show that R.T. with, I think, Waldo the Magician. (R.T. Notes read: *pt appeared to enjoy himself—he smiled!* However, I was just smiling at the blonde, not really enjoying the show.) I started to talk to a young man and young woman there who were both quite physically disabled and discovered that they had the same feelings about this place: they wanted to get out as much as I did. Realizing that I was not the only one with such feelings made me a little more social but I still resisted attending group events. Not everyone was easy to get along with, especially the patients with head injuries. No one told me much about the other patients, so I never realized why they were having so much difficulty. Several had head injuries without noticeable physical disabilities and I could not understand why they had such a hard time getting around.

When a recreational therapist asked me to go to the movies where *ET* was playing, I told her that it was a movie I had no interest in, but in reality I was terrified to go out. We were going to take another person with us and I didn't want to be seen in public in my less-than-capable state, let alone with another patient from this awful place. But the young lady who was going smiled at me and I went along with her and the therapist like an obedient puppy dog. I loved the movie and became very good friends with the young lady as well.

Soon I received passes to go home for the weekend—almost as if this were a prison and I was allowed out for good behavior. It was fantastic to get a good home-cooked dinner and be with friends and family, but all too soon came Sunday night and I had to go back. I felt that it was inhumane, that I was being punished for a crime I hadn't committed. I pleaded with my mother to let me stay home but I finally learned that I had to play by the rules and respect the recovery process. It still felt like I was a small kid who had been told to be good or he would never go home.

(Shawn's mother has a far different memory. She remembers that he was scared to come home. She says he was so afraid to be without the structure and the support of the hospital staff that he would beg to be allowed to return almost as soon as he arrived.)

Occupational therapy was part of the process and my therapist was a lady named Patty Plummer. She was fun; a great listener and not only knew her job, but knew how to get me to work. Whatever challenge she had for me, I tried to find a way to get around it. She had asked my mother to bring in a shirt with buttons, but I couldn't line up those darned buttons so I wanted to solve the problem by wearing T-shirts. Patty had ways for making me let my guard down and get me to make an attempt by telling me jokes. I accepted the fact that I was lucky and finally I did get that shirt buttoned, but we agreed that T-shirts would be more convenient for now.

Patty Plummer, OT, reminisces that, due to my initial impairments, I did not understand the full extent of my stroke.

He was impulsive, severely disabled and lacked insight. He wanted to walk before he could sit up straight for example, and he usually did not understand the reason we had to work on self-care skills when he thought he could do them himself, which he couldn't. He was focused on a full return of function in his left arm. I was always impressed how he did not give up, so perhaps some of his lack of awareness was a good thing. His recovery was long term, as it always is after a stroke. After discharge from Rehab it appeared he was not always careful to follow the recommended plan, but he was young and wanted to take chances. In retrospect, that seems like a great thing! I was impressed again with his tenacity to procure a job at MMC, go to school and continue his activities, such as playing pool, etc., despite the loss of function in his left arm and what appeared to be high level cognitive defects.

At some point I began cooking-on a real stove—a little dangerous, I thought, but just what I needed. I could understand the practicality of this, especially as we were making cheeseburgers. Cutting food and eating it however, was a challenge. Patty brought me a rocker knife that was a joke. It wasn't sharp enough to butter bread and I was supposed to rock it back and forth! There were also these devices to assist me to slip on shoes or to tie shoelaces one-handed and even a block of wood to hold playing cards. I hated all of them. They were made for cripples, not me! These little gadgets angered me so I told Patty that, if these were the best the medical field could come up with, they stank. I could do better myself.

Patty, more than anyone else in the hospital, knew when I needed to let my frustrations out, and she took me into the testing lab. This place was part of the kitchen and I hated it with a passion. I felt like a test rat there, picking up little foam blocks or fitting things together and always being timed. This time she gave me a basket full of beanbags. "Throw them as hard as you can at anything you want," she told me. Bad idea, Pat! She didn't realize just how strong I was and how angry. She had left the kitchen door open and the first bag went flying out, barely missing someone passing by. The second and third smashed well outside in the corridor making a very loud noise. Patty had to shut the door quickly as I continued to hurl those bags. It felt really awesome to do that. Pat was my hero then and still is my hero today, but we never got to play that game again.

In those days, rehabilitation was in its infancy and I was not in a very receptive state of mind either. To any disabled person who is entering rehab now in the twenty-first century, I must tell you that rehab has progressed to reflect the way our society has changed its attitude towards the disabled. Physical, occupational, recreational and vocational therapists who were working then and are still working now will attest to the fact that back in the '80s the goal of rehabilitation was to enable the patient to be discharged from the hospital to live at home, independently or not, as the case may be. Today the goal is to get the patient back into society as a functioning, effective member of the community. I can state this as fact, but I know that to any person who is entering that unknown territory, it is little consolation for the harsh reality of having your whole life changed so suddenly and drastically by a physical event.

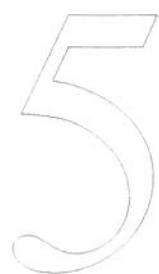

Home

Courage is the price that life exacts
for granting peace.

Amelia Earhart, from Courage

I was told about a week before, that on August 27th I was to be discharged. I couldn't wait!—or could I? It was like being a kid at Christmas, but on the other hand, I wasn't 100% sure of myself. I had been away for what seemed to be a long time; I still had a bad limp and my fingers didn't work the way they used to. I had a lot of doubts, which was new and strange to me as I had always been so self-confident before my stroke.

Back when I graduated from High School in 1981, I used to go fishing with my father and brother. Those were some of the best times of my life. I got to know them both better as we worked those long, brutal hours, sharing the great adventure of learning more about the sea, and I grew up quickly. It was tough work and it made me tough. As a kid with heart trouble, I couldn't play aerobic sports such as running track or basketball, but lifting weights was easy. Still, for me the best thing was being with friends; going to the beach and the lakes-boating, tubing and swimming, leading the active, confident life.

So now I started to get a little panicky. I was always so physically fit before the stroke, but afterward everything had changed. Nevertheless, I remembered that I had survived this hell and everything should be gravy from now on. The staff at the hospital had done their best to help me recover and now it was up to me. I would be doing outpatient therapy, which meant I would have to be tough and do what I had always done: work hard to get back in shape. But I wasn't sure what I could do with my limitations.

All this had been as hard on the family as it had been for me. However, here it was at last, the day of my discharge . . . my dad and uncle were on their way.

When Dad came in, I could see he was trying to put on a strong face as always. I didn't know which one of us was more nervous, Dad or me. Uncle

George, however, wore a big smirk as he said, "Let's get out of here!" That sounded great to me. He had been there for me from the beginning and I'll never forget that. Dad and Uncle George were tough men and I wanted to be the same and show no fear, yet I always got this warm feeling from them both. I could feel their love. I asked my dad where my mother was and he told me that she was getting the house ready for me.

My mother had been advised by the social worker to apply for SSI and SSDI for me. She was also told that she would need to be home with me for about three weeks, depending on when she felt I would be ready to stay at home alone. So my mother arranged to take a leave of absence from her job as manager of a pharmacy. She said she felt confident that she could manage, and she did.

When I arrived home, I felt like a prisoner who had just been released. I felt joyous but still a little uncertain, but it was the best day of my life because I was with my family again. They were as nervous as I was, and I could tell my mother was nervous too, as she was busy running around the house. All in all it was a great day to be alive, and I knew deep inside that this had been a close one for me.

Dear Shawn,

I guess I can't say that I know how you must feel, because I've never been through it. There is one thing I do know, that is, that you are the strongest person I know. You always say you can take anyone that comes along. This is not a someone that you have to beat, it is a "something". But if something can be beat, we all know "you can beat it! Just like having a long bout with someone, this is going to take time, but if you believe in yourself, and your strength, you can do anything in the world. We all love you more than anything in the world, and we're all behind you 100%. You have millions of friends and a bunch of family to call on. We won't let anything happen to you. Just do me one favor, get better and (well, two) SMILE!!!

I LOVE YOU
VERY, VERY,
MUCH

love,
Kathi

Letter from Kathi

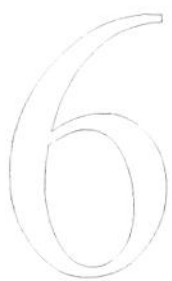

Kathi's Story

The world breaks everyone
and afterward many are strong
at the broken places.
But those that will not break, it kills.

Ernest Hemingway,
from a A Farewell to Arms

Kathi is my younger sister. Here is her version of the story.

—

I haven't thought about this for . . . well, I guess I never did let myself think about that day. I'm not sure where in my memories it has been hiding, but for some reason it has chosen now to emerge from the shadows: the day I lost one brother—at least in body—

and gained another quite entirely. Not by death, but by a change intended by some Greater Force.

It was a typically boring summer day for this then 14-year old, and I had decided I would go roller-skating. As I tackled the dirt and rock road from our house, Shawn's friend Todd was on his way down in his Corvette or whatever it was. Todd lived with us at the time so it wasn't so unusual to see him—what was unusual was the look on his face. He looked like he was in shock; really scared and I remember feeling scared, too—when you just know something is wrong before you know.

Frantic, he shouted, "Where's your mother and father—go get them! Where are they?" That's all I remember about that moment. I don't even know now if Todd said it was Shawn or not, I just remember the sheer panic. Who went to the hospital? How? When? All I know is I did not know. . . .

Shannon, my niece, was just a new baby and I stayed home and cared for her so that my brother Jeff and his wife, Beth, could go to the hospital. Oddly, if I remember correctly (and now having preteens of my own, I understand) I couldn't wrap my brain around the fact that something tragic had happened to anyone close to me; my biggest concern at the moment was baby-sitting a very fussy baby.

I don't know when I was told what happened. I know Mom and Dad and Jeff and Beth were always at the hospital, but I don't know at what point what had happened was explained to me. I have no recollection of feeling the true force of this tragedy and what it meant for my brother, but I got some idea of what it would mean to my family one night at dinner.

It wasn't even a whole night that stuck with me, but one single moment: an amazingly sad, sickening moment. Mom, Dad, and I went to a local restaurant for dinner. The restaurant itself was wicked dark and empty. We were sitting at this depressing little table in the dark and I can still see my mother's face. It was blank. I wonder now if she was in shock, considering how close it was to the actual day this happened. My father, my big, burly, tough-as-nails dad, was helpless at that moment. He sat with his head in his hands, something I'd only seen him do in the quiet of an early morning when he thought he was alone, so I knew he was scared. I don't know what I thought then or what I knew. In the background there was music playing: Kermit the Frog's rendition of Rainbow Connection. I cannot hear that song to this day without seeing that scene or feeling that moment all over again.

I'm trying to put things in some chronological order, but I cannot. I think I was removed enough from the nucleus of all that was going on that my memories are in bits and pieces. But if I had to say what order this next memory came, it would have to be fairly soon after Shawn had the stroke because I'm sure I was asking questions and wanting to see him. My mother did take me to the hospital, how often I don't recall, but this particular day I remember. It does seem as if it was my first time—and you can well imagine the images I'd created in my mind based on what little information I'd received on his condition. It was a beautiful day and we were going to take Shawn out on some sort of roof or to a solarium-type room. Of course he was in a wheelchair and the only other 'difference' I recall was his slurred speech. I remember he seemed to go in and out of confusion pretty easily, and I also remember a conversation about who had been in to see him and the big surprise that all his friends and acquaintances had been in except his very best friend, Dave Tonneson. We were all so surprised and as it turns out, it was a long time I think before he ever did go in. See, another random memory.

Despite the lack of any humor in what had happened to my brother, there were moments that were, well . . . funny. Shawn absolutely hated my dog Mitzi—almost as much as he hated his pre-teen sister. I was always scared I would come home one day to find my dog hanging from a tree . . . Shawn's temper was famous. So I was surprised when one day he asked my mother if she could bring Mitzi into the hospital to see him, saying he missed her! But that bizarre loss of memory wasn't so funny when my poor mom would get home every evening exhausted, physically and emotionally, from a day in the hospital with Shawn, and no sooner would she walk through the door than the phone would ring. "Why haven't you been in to see me?" Shawn would say. "When are you coming to see me?" Already he'd forgotten.

I had a boyfriend, my first boyfriend and at 14 couldn't ask for more than to spend a day with him. One day my mother had asked his mother if I could join him and his family on the beach, which was a short walk from our house. This day I remember because I just couldn't make myself enjoy it. I felt a panic in my chest that I'm not sure I could have explained then, let alone now. I walked home. Actually, I'm pretty sure I ran. My mother of course was at the hospital, but I must have felt some urgency to be close to home.

When Shawn was able to come home for overnights or later on weekends, it gradually became very apparent to me that my brother would never be the same. Neither would any of our lives. To be honest, it was never very enjoyable to have him home. I say this for a lot of reasons but mostly for what I felt I thought was his embarrassment and loss of humility. Whether or not he had the ability to conceptualize those things in his stroke-altered brain, I don't know. I knew that when he needed to be helped to the bathroom (actually getting there was a long, involved process), or needed help to eat his meals, he must, as a young, formerly healthy 20-year-old, feel awfully bad inside. I couldn't stand watching it. And when my mother and father had an actual argument over the black, rubber-handled, special utensils, I knew it would be a very, very long road for Shawn. My mom was cutting up Shawn's meat with these horribly awkward black, spongy-handled utensils and my father was yelling at her because the whole purpose of these implements was to allow Shawn to do it himself. Shawn hated them, and that was the beginning of the formation of the kind of man he is today.

He was not handicapped even if he was very much so. He was determined to find ways of doing things that were 'normal.' I'm not sure which was worse, having Shawn come home for the day or having to take him back to the hospital at night. Which was more heartbreaking—watching him struggle or leaving him at night all alone in his hospital room to think about it? It was gut-wrenching.

When Shawn finally came home to stay we had to put his room, which had been in the basement, upstairs. My father had rigged up this whole pulley system for some sort of exercises for Shawn, and to me it seemed Shawn spent a great deal of his time in that room; whether he was exercising or crying, I'll never know. Whatever he was doing, it was the beginning of a road for my brother that brought him challenges and successes that some other young man would have avoided like big orange road blocks. Not Shawn. If he didn't have enough challenge, he created it. Not only did he learn to adapt to daily living, he was gunned up for new beginnings. He went back to school. I would have never believed that the brother I "hated"—never got along with—would be sitting at the kitchen table begging me to teach him math facts. Not physics, but addition and subtraction, multiplication and division, all over again. Basics . . . he had to go back to basics. I didn't think he could succeed at what he was striving for (I think at the time he was attending some night school classes so that he could then take an ECG reading class, but I'm not sure). But I am sure I was not the only one who doubted. We saw his daily struggles . . . DAILY struggles. I have to chuckle now because he showed us in so many ways how he was succeeding but we couldn't see it at the time.

Shawn fought harder and worked harder than anyone could imagine—not just to "get back what he lost" but to be more of a person than he probably would have been had he not suffered his tragedy.

This is my mother's memory; I've only heard it, I never had to go through the witnessing of it, but it's something I often think about when Shawn enjoys a new accomplishment in his life. She talks about the day the physical therapist insisted that she come in and watch Shawn's therapy. Now, it must have been in mom's mind that she was going to see him get up and try to walk—you know, just like TV stories when the patient is up on the parallel bars and takes those first miraculous steps. No! What my mother got to see was her 20-year-old son learn to crawl. And that was a big day. That perhaps was the pivotal moment for my mother. She must have been struck as if by an eighteen-wheeler with the fact that her son, as she had known him, was gone. There in front of her was someone she didn't know, and her life fell apart then . . . although not for long. My mother readied herself, too, for the new road, but in those moments it must have gone spinning out of control for her, perhaps more so than in the seconds when she learned of the stroke itself.

I think about that memory and where Shawn is now. I think about all the times he tried to do all the things he used to be able to do, like skiing. Or even just wearing cowboy boots. Maybe he figured out in his own time that either he couldn't do them, or he just didn't want to do them any more, and he moved on. Not merely forward but in the most incredible ways, and that is why I'm so honored to be a part of his life. He is truly a hero, not the kind that flies, but the kind that rescues people, people like himself that have lost and are lost. He gives them back some dignity, or maybe he just shows them where to find it: within themselves.

Part ll

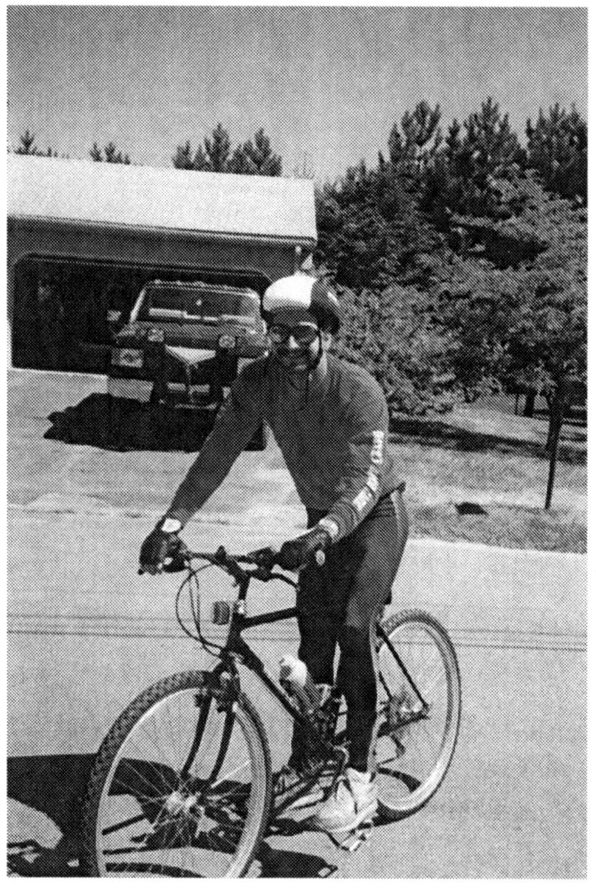

After the stroke

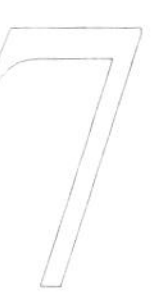

Recovery and Discovery

In the confrontation between stream and rock
the stream always wins—not because of
strength,
but because of persistence

Anonymous

My disability made me feel very vulnerable, especially after being used to being so strong and able-bodied. Now my left side worked marginally at best, and I could barely walk, let alone defend myself. Going down stairs without railings was immensely difficult, as railings were uncommon then; this was long before the Americans with Disabilities Act was passed. Likewise walking on uneven ground, because my balance was so unsure. I still had to attend rehab at the hospital three times a week, but it was then I realized that from now on recovery was really up to me.

—

Jeanette, Shawn's mother remembers:

When he finally was discharged, self-conscious, he refused to go out. Patty Stogsdill, one of his [physical therapists] . . . finally came and got him and forced him to go to a party with some other PTs.

There was a doctor who wrote a letter stating that Shawn was 'borderline'-would never be any better; that he covered by making up what he couldn't remember. Shawn, his father and I were very angry when we received this letter and this letter fueled Shawn's determination to get better at any cost. Two years later, Shawn had a job at Maine Medical Center and had to take courses. He memorized hundreds of drugs. I sent the results to the doctor who had written the note telling us he was fit for nothing!

—

I started with stretching and crunches to build up my strength then moved on to weights, light ones at first, 5 and 10 pounds. Next came walking. I walked everywhere. At that time my family lived by Crescent Beach State Park in Cape Elizabeth which has a great, curving sandy beach about one mile long. I started to walk a loop along the beach a little at a time, until finally I was making the whole two-mile loop. I then began walking slowly without the cane, keeping it with me just in case I got into trouble. I played with it, whipping it around while thinking of ways to use it to protect myself if needed. (At that time, I had no clue where this casual start would lead me.) All I had was a metal cane and it finally broke when I was whipping it around on the beach and struck a rock. The bottom half went out to sea so I just walked more and more without it. I was learning that recovery was all about persistence—never giving up.

My parents bought me some push-up bars so that was added to my routine of chin-ups with both hands. Every day I did a little more and when I became competent with chin-ups, I began one-armed pull-ups. My brother, Jeff, couldn't do as many as I could and that secretly made me feel very good. My father told me that I would wear out every part of my body if I didn't slow down, but I knew it was his way of telling me I was doing a good job.

Relearning to ride a bicycle was one of my toughest activities. The bicycle was my sister's and the surface was our dirt driveway. I fell, spilling quite a little blood, as I was on anti-coagulants, and earning several scars on my arms and legs. After the wounds healed and my walking and balance improved I tried again, realizing that learning to ride had become a proving point for me. I rode about 10 feet and caught myself before I fell. I hadn't been able to do that before as my right leg had not been so strong. The next time I managed to ride the entire 40-foot length of the driveway. It felt great! I knew that I had done all I could with this bike and I needed a better one. Mountain bikes were becoming more popular and all my friends were biking off-road, so I bought an excellent mountain bike from one of them, mastered it and began to bike constantly. I usually did master whatever I attempted but not always on the first try. I was stubborn and failure was never an option.

I still hung out with my friends but my interests were rather different from theirs as I was much more focused upon healthy living. They still enjoyed partying but I had lost my taste for it. I was still very self-conscious about the way I looked when I went out in public and stayed away from crowded areas as much as possible.

In 1983, my family moved to the other side of Cape Elizabeth, and there I started to lift weights in earnest. I was given a new 250 lb. set of iron weights for Christmas and I remember my father helping me to set it up. He thought I was crazy to attempt to lift this much weight, but I was getting quite built-up and always trying to improve myself. I was now addicted to exercise and had to have it every day. All this weightlifting and biking were making my legs stronger and I was getting better as well as looking better, so I went out more often with my friends. They were always looking out for me and didn't pressure me to drink. I was comfortable with people who knew me, knew what had happened and didn't treat me as if I had three heads. We played hard, going to my friend Dave's camp to water-ski and tube. I even went to the shooting range and did very well there and also tried shooting pool. Patty Plummer, who was still my occupational therapist, made me a brace for my left hand so I could steady the cue. I still have it today.

I loved to swim and, even if I had trouble getting back in the boat, there was always someone to help me. My friends seemed to know instinctively how much to help me and when to let me do things on my own. They knew I didn't want any special favors. When we went out to eat, they would let me know if I had food left on my face and one would tap the side of his face to make me aware and wipe my face.

None of them had any idea just how dangerous it was for me to do all this fun stuff such as tubing, rope-swinging or biking. I knew that the rehab staff wanted me to take fewer chances due to the fact that I could bleed to death as I had to take a rather large dose of blood thinner (Coumadin) daily in order to avoid another stroke. If I should go out one night and have a couple of beers, it would wreak havoc on my blood clotting as alcohol interacts with Coumadin and increases its anticoagulant effect on the blood. In retrospect, I didn't display the best judgment. I had no plans to slow down as the stroke itself had caused me to slow down much more than I wanted.

One night I went out with my friends and had a couple of drinks. When I got home, I had a really heavy nosebleed. My parents found a trail of blood from the door to the bathroom as well as all the bloody tissues in the wastebasket when they got up in the morning, and it scared them. I realized then that it was time to grow up and become a responsible adult. I had had all the fun I needed and more, and I was not getting any younger. My doctors and my parents were telling me the same thing. I needed and more and I was not getting any younger. My doctors and my parents were telling me the same thing. I had already been forced to grow up a lot by the stroke but, up until now, something in my mind just didn't want to focus on that fact. Each time I went to outpatient rehabilitation it was obvious that I needed it less and less, so they sent me to vocational rehab for help to return to work.

Exercising and playing had become a little boring. You can only bike or walk so many miles and I finally had peaked at weightlifting when I bench-pressed 265 lbs. That tore my rotator cuff and I had to have surgery to fix it, so my father was right. Except for the left-sided weakness I was physically in great shape. I needed a new adventure. However, when I reflect back on the time off I had after the stroke, I realize that I was extremely lucky as all I had to worry about was getting myself back in shape. I had had time to be alone to reflect on my life and ponder what I wanted to do with it. Most people never get that chance.

Vocational rehabilitation evaluated me and they didn't believe I would do well in college at that time. (I would never forget that and later would prove them wrong.) I couldn't do the outdoors work that I had always enjoyed before the stroke, so it was decided that I should try a job in the hospital.

When I was a kid, I had been in and out of hospitals for my cardiac tests and had always wanted to work in one, so I applied to Pediatrics as a nursing assistant/unit helper. I started work on June 16, 1984, 23 months after the stroke. I stocked shelves and made sure that each room had the supplies it needed. It was a great job with which to begin my new working career, but it was a tough unit; so heartbreaking to see all those very sick little kids with their worried families. I was happy to help out by doing whatever I could for them. This helped me to grow up. I took my job very seriously; I didn't make much money but it was what I did that counted and it was good to be able to give back what I had received from the caring health professionals at Maine Medical Center. Everything that I experienced at the hospital, both the good and the bad, helped me to learn and grow.

—

Dr. Sullivan reminisces:

In the two years after the stroke, [while Shawn was] enduring some difficult therapy and trying to come to terms with the effects of the stroke, I witnessed an amazing transformation as Shawn grew up and became a responsible adult. I remember Shawn working at MMC for years as a cardiology technician. He was always cheerful and efficient, adapting his disability to his duties amazingly well.

—

Determined to do the best job possible, I learned a great deal about children from the patients as well as the parents, nurses and doctors on Pediatrics. I had to go to other departments as well to obtain supplies for my unit, so I gained more experience interacting with different people.

After a year and a half, I had gone as far as I could in that job and it was time to move on.

I enjoyed working at the hospital and wanted more responsibility. There was an opening in Cardiology as a ECG technician and I applied and was accepted. I was leaving a familiar place where I had become comfortable to try something new but I was learning that in order to grow and change, I had to constantly challenge myself.

It was not an easy job and definitely was a challenge, but I adapted and learned quickly. I was a fast study, and in those days on-the-job training was considered the most important learning method. I was started out slowly on stable, easy patients for the first week or so. I had some difficulty using the equipment as it wasn't meant to be operated one-handed but I was fortunate, as new equipment was just becoming available when I began work in Cardiology. My supervisor was progressive and we tried out a lot of the new equipment. For instance, I was the only person to use some new leads for the ECG cart because they were so expensive, but I discovered they were very user-friendly for the one-handed. Working there was difficult and challenging as I had to do everything with my right hand, but learning to adapt every technique needed on the equipment gave me great confidence in my abilities.

I remember my first code: I was sent into a room full of people trying to revive a person in dire straits. Everyone moved out of the way to let me do the ECG. There was quite a bit of pressure to do it quickly, efficiently and one-handed with fifteen people looking over my shoulder impatiently. I discovered that I functioned well under pressure and grew to like it.

I never knew what I would face on any given day. I went to every department and nursing unit in the hospital and saw many different as well as difficult medical situations, which made me a much stronger person. Georgann Dicky, still an RN on R4, remembers seeing her former patient, now a colleague, when I tested a patient on her floor, told me I was doing splendidly. Patty Stogsdill M.D. (who used to be one of my physical therapists, and is now my physician and a longtime friend) says that I was always smiling when I worked as an ECG tech and, even though I was one-handed, I just improvised and did my job efficiently. I always strove to be the best I could be.

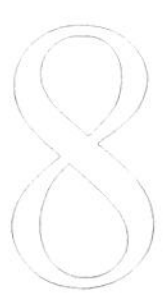

Marriage and College

There is no more lovely, friendly and charming
relationship . . . than a good marriage.

Martin Luther, from Table Talk

When I was working in Cardiology, I met a very good-looking nurse with a strange sense of humor. Extremely intelligent and knowledgeable on many subjects, Andrea seemed to follow the beat of a different drummer; she was flexible enough to change with her environment when needed, but stuck firmly to her principles and beliefs. She offered to take me out to Tortilla Flats, a Portland Mexican restaurant, for my birthday. We hit it off and have been together ever since. I had done all the playing I wanted to do and was ready to meet the right person. She changed my life greatly for the better, and

I consider her to be my better half, my partner both in life and in business, and it is because of her that I have developed and changed in so many ways.

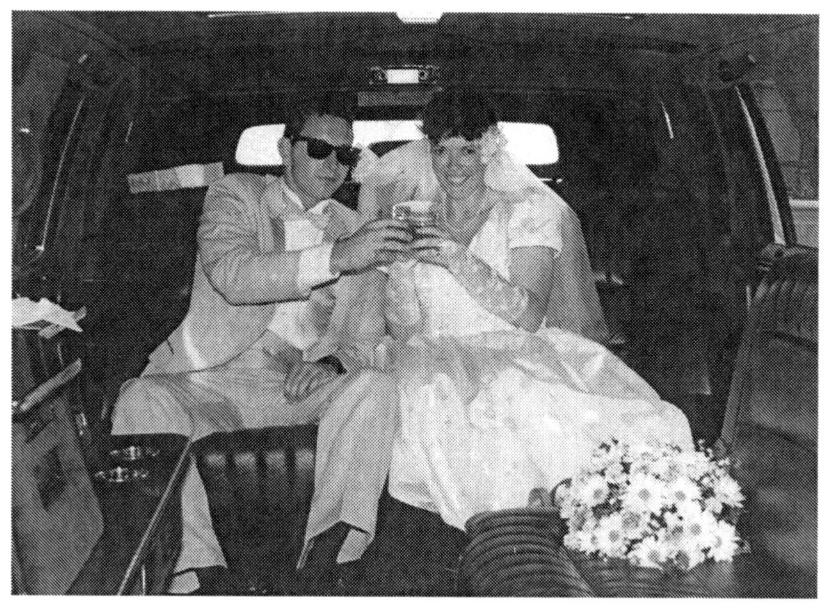

Shawn and Andrea's Wedding Day – July 20, 1991

Andrea says: "Shawn is my best friend and soul mate. He accepts my insanity and, no matter how angry we get with each other, at the end of the day we want to be together."

Although we didn't have much money and little experience, I think we did a great job of planning the wedding ourselves. I remember spending hours with

Andrea one night making what seemed to me to be a million table favors—little plastic glasses, netting and pastel M & Ms. I had a few choice words to say but Andrea just smiled and said that this was bringing us closer together.

We were married July 20, 1991, on one of the hottest days of a very long heat wave. It was 98 degrees at noon and it felt as if I was in a sauna in my tuxedo. Guests changed into shorts and swimsuits at the reception in Cape Elizabeth. There were a lot of people and we had fun dancing with many fans running to try to beat the heat. We honeymooned in New Hampshire at my friend Dave's camp that thankfully was on a lake, as the heat continued. To end a great week, people converged on the camp to celebrate Dave's birthday.

After working for 10 years in the medical field I needed a change of pace, so, in the fall of 1994, I went back to school at Husson College in Portland, conveniently just down the hill from the hospital. I had always felt cheated by the stroke that prevented me from going to college after high school, but in reality it had only been postponed. I was now working full-time and going to school part-time which allowed me to work at my own pace. I did well, always getting

A's and B's even though I had to work hard and needed a tutor for some courses as it had been a long time since I was a student. Even when it was tough I believed that it was important to stick it out. I became a business major as I wanted to start my own business someday and to work for myself, and I knew I needed education and a strong foundation to help me run it. I was not the greatest accounting student, but I did learn how to read a balance sheet. I enjoyed the public speaking class. The teacher was superb and I learned a great deal from the course that I now use every day when teaching my classes. Economics was also enjoyable and learning how to run a business was fun and I was certain that the knowledge would be useful in the future.

But life wasn't all hard work. Andrea and I had taken up hiking in the early '90s and spent many of our summer vacations camping and hiking in the White Mountains of New Hampshire and in Acadia National Park. It was a great way to get outside and experience nature as well as stay in shape. We thoroughly enjoyed hiking through the forests and among the mountains far away from noise and technology. After a while on the trail, we even forgot the bugs. At night, sitting around a campfire, we reveled in the scent of burning wood—far better than any $100-an-ounce perfume, and it kept the mosquitos at bay! It was magical, mesmerizing to watch the campfire sizzle and snap, sending sparks flying. Away from the city lights, the night skies were crystal clear and the stars shone brighter than any gemstone. We survived thunderstorms when we had to dig trenches to prevent our tent from being flooded, squirrel attacks and hungry, biting insects, and learned the art of cooking masterpieces on a tabletop grill.

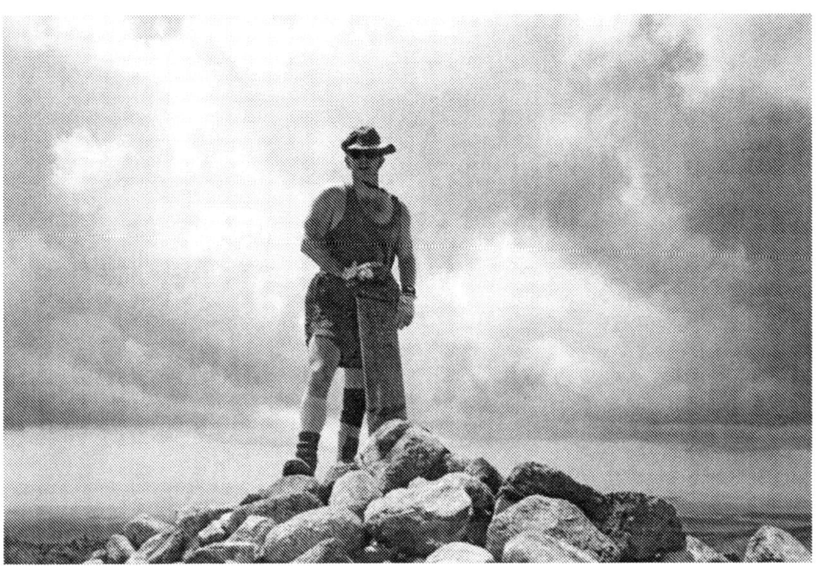

One summer we climbed Tuckerman's Ravine on Mount Washington, the tallest mountain in New

England. It was one of those rare summer days when the weather was perfect, the sky beautifully clear and bright blue. It took us eight hours for the round trip and it was a little disappointing to get to the top and be greeted by the hundred or so tourists browsing the gift shops who had driven up the auto road. But it is the journey, not the goal that brings you the most pleasure.

On one of our trips to Acadia National Park on Mount Desert Island, we decided to try a different and more difficult trail than any we had previously hiked. We had always wanted to do the Precipice Trail—described in the trail guide as "very steep, exposed cliffs and ledges, with iron rungs and ladders"—but as usual at that time of year (early summer) it was closed because peregrine falcons were nesting near that trail. We were told that the Beehive Trail near Sandy Beach was similar in difficulty: "Woods to exposed cliffs, iron rungs on ledges." We started up the mountain. It didn't look bad from the bottom. There was a sign that marked it as difficult and dangerous . . . but who looks at signs? It was a nice day, yet in the first half-hour we saw several people turning back. So far the trail wasn't bad so we continued to climb. Then it got steep—suddenly. The path, two feet wide in good areas, worked its way along a rock face. Andrea went ahead of me to scout out the climb ahead. I crawled across a very narrow little wooden bridge and from then on, my back was against the rock as the trail had narrowed to match the width of the bridge. I kept asking Andrea if it was getting better up ahead and she replied, "Not really," but at that point we thought we had gone too far to turn back. Hoping that we were almost done, we came to some large iron rungs that went around a very big rock. They would have been a challenge for most climbers but for a person with only one arm it was nearly impossible! I had to jump from one rung to the next with a deadly drop if I missed it.

Andrea was becoming more and more concerned about my safety but I told her that I couldn't go back. Each new turn in the trail seemed to come with more rungs and more challenges. My right arm was bleeding from hitting the rocks when I lunged to catch the next rung. I imagined that someone with a perverse sense of humor had removed every other rung just to increase the difficulty. Every time Andrea went around a corner, I would again ask her if it was getting better and again she would reply, "Not really." Finally we reached the top and opted to come down on an easier trail at the back of the mountain. Oh, yes: the view of the ocean from the top was incredible! I am eternally grateful for the peregrine falcons. If they hadn't been nesting, we probably would have tried the Precipice instead, listed as more difficult than the Beehive!

We were living a full life. My self image was much better. I was back in full force, doing what I had wanted to do for a long time, and it felt great.

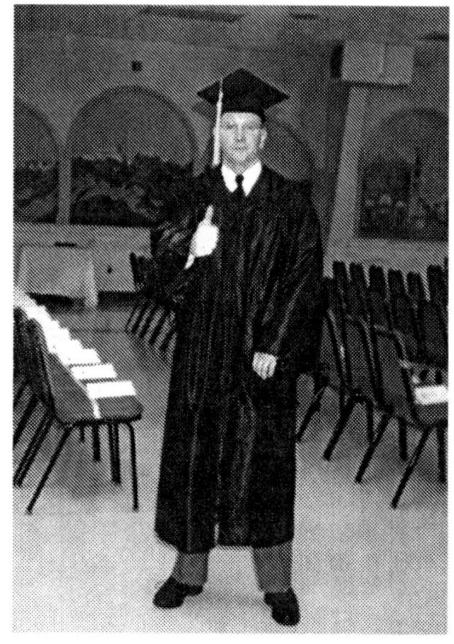

Graduation from Husson College - 2000

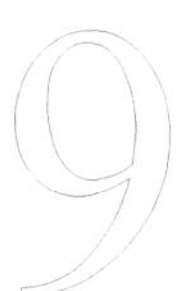

Martial Arts

Hold yourself responsible for a higher standard
than anyone else expects of you.
Never excuse yourself.

Henry Ward Beecher

One of the biggest things Andrea and I share is our love for the martial arts that we both began to study three years after we met and married. Eventually we decided to make it one of our lives' vocations because of all that it has given us, and we wanted to give back what we had been given.

While I was attending college, although I was married and working full-time in addition to my studies, I still had great difficulty with my left arm and leg. I thought that some form of formal exercise might be helpful. Near the hospital, in the building next to my college, there was a martial arts school called Masters of Self-defense. I had always wanted to learn martial arts after watching Kung Fu in movies such as *Billy Jack* and Bruce Lee's *Enter the Dragon.* My curiosity got the better of me, even if I wasn't sure if I could handle martial arts as well as work and school, but (as is obvious by now) I always enjoyed a challenge. One day in the fall of 1994, I asked Andrea to come with me to check out the school. Although she was reluctant, she knew that I really wanted to go. She was fascinated with martial arts and action movies, but didn't think it would be possible to study them herself. We went with no idea of what to expect, even though we had friends who had taken martial arts and loved it.

As we entered the door of the school—which felt like a huge step in itself—we were met in the lobby by a bald man wearing a black *gi* who was about my age. More than anything else, I remember his eyes, because as we talked about martial arts they seemed to light up. He didn't attempt to sell us anything; he answered my questions and told me that he thought it would be good for me. We didn't sign up that day as the master of the school was not in. The person that we met was Peter Jordan, and as we talked we realized that we knew many of the same people. Peter would eventually become my chief instructor and remains one of my closest friends to this day.

Both Andrea and I agreed to give martial arts a try. Meeting Peter was a positive step, and then we met the owner of the school, Master Inman, who also ran it. He too had that sparkle in his eyes and an obvious passion for what he was doing. My only disappointment was finding out the Master taught mostly day classes, as I had to take evening classes to fit in with my work and college schedule.

We began with a private class held by a pleasant woman who was a third-degree brown belt. She taught us some kicks and punches to get us ready for our first class. My balance was not good and I nearly landed on my rear attempting my first kick, but managed to save myself from falling and looking stupid. I thought the instructor would laugh, but she smiled in sympathy and told me that she had never been well-coordinated either, and when she first started she had lost her balance too. That made me feel better. Both Andrea (who did much better than I did) and I liked all the people we met. Everyone had a positive attitude and seemed confident in themselves.

After that first session we started classes on September 12, 1994, and immediately it seemed to me that this was something that I had been looking for right from the day I left rehab. Andrea also liked it. Our schedules weren't the same so we didn't get to all the classes together. Those beginning classes were not hard because the instructors took it slowly at first. Usually one of the brown belt instructors would warm up the class with the kicking and punching techniques that were taught to all the students. I, however, began to get a little frustrated as sometimes I had to wait to have them adapted to my abilities.

I was always early for evening classes. Right after work I would come in and talk to Master Inman. He was always willing to answer the million-and-one questions I had—as long as it was before class. Once class started it was time to focus and learn. He told me that I should leave everything outside the Dojo and just focus on the present: practicing my martial arts. Nothing else should exist in that time. It was very difficult to do so for the first month or so as I always had to wait to get instructions to adapt a technique so Master Inman suggested that I take some private instruction in order to keep up with the class.

By now I was hooked and determined to stick this out and so was Andrea. This was something we could do together year-round; something that we could also take out of the Dojo and practice at home. I did think of giving up a few times but studying together helped us both to keep focused. Together we pushed ourselves and challenged each other to get off the couch when going to class was too great an effort. We were each other's crowbar, as Andrea liked to say.

She always knew which buttons to push to keep me going, so I started private lessons with Master Inman. They took much of the frustration away and gave me confidence, as some of the techniques I learned were better than the ones the class learned. We worked so hard for the first couple of months getting ready to test: practice, practice, practice. Kicks and punches at least a thousand times and more. I learned that Master Inman was well known in the area for developing some of the best students around. It took a lot of hard training and tough discipline, which I began to develop.

Andrea and I began to study martial arts at the same time as many other people started and we soon noticed that one by one, they dropped out. Many of those whom I considered talented and much better than I was didn't even make to the first rank: yellow belt. We were told from the beginning that those who would last would be those who wanted it the most.

"Cream always rises to the top," Sensei Peter Jordan had said.

Sticking with it was a badge of toughness in itself. The instructors and the master were hard on everyone; no slacking off allowed. Pushups were meted out for the slightest infraction such as walking into the Dojo with street shoes on.

I didn't want any special favors—and I didn't get any. I enjoyed the fact that no one was easy on me: I was expected to work as hard as everyone else. I didn't do a great job kicking and I wasn't the most graceful student, but I was one of the students most determined to make it through the kenpo program. Once we had done a drill a million times (that's what it felt like), such as kicking up and down the Dojo in the kenpo "half-mooning" walking technique, we then moved on to another drill that was harder. After six weeks I noticed that my stamina was better; I didn't get as winded and I didn't break out into a sweat as easily as I did at the beginning. My balance had improved and my will to do better was getting stronger with every class. Of course, my muscles were sore from each workout and sometimes I was frustrated, but the master always knew what to say to make us tough it out and keep going. To get a "good job!" out of him required a Herculean effort from everyone including me. He made us do each technique over and over until we were able to perform it perfectly. As the weeks and the months progressed, most of the students we started with dropped out one by one as new students joined. It was encouraging in a way to know that we were surviving where others could not.

—

Peter Jordan:

I remember Shawn and Andrea when they came into the Masters of Self-Defence Dojo to inquire about studying martial arts. I was one of Master Inman's Instructors and was in the lobby when they came in. Shawn was certainly not as muscled or built-up and as confident as he is now. He struck me as very eager, very curious.

Master Inman was 'old school'; he believed in the old, hard way of teaching martial arts, with absolutely no exceptions. "You do it again and again and again until you get it right. You do pushups for the slightest infraction of the Dojo rules," etc. He did tend to have the "favorite student of the week" and you always knew who it was. I don't think that he was extra hard on Shawn in particular, as Shawn was so determined to learn, took private lessons and tried so hard.

—

Master Inman was going to test students for their next rank on November 4, 1994. If we passed, Andrea and I would no longer be white belts, which would feel good. Testing in martial arts was both physically and mentally challenging while maintaining safety. We were put in various situations to see if we could think on our feet and react appropriately. We didn't know what to expect and were apprehensive when we showed up in full *gi* for the test, but I have since learned it is that unknown that keeps you alert at all times!

A few people who had started with us were testing for their yellow belts too but there were also students present going for higher ranks. They didn't seem any less nervous than we were.

We stood in a line in Front Position: feet together, knees slightly bent, one hand in a fist with the other open to cover the fist, eyes focused forward—the traditional stance for bowing, greeting other martial artists, or getting ready for class. In kenpo karate, the fist represents power, and the open hand, control: power is meaningless without control.

Master Inman came out with his test face on. We could tell this was not going to be easy. The test started with basics: kicks and strikes for what felt like hours. I messed up a little as I was so nervous and that is just why the test was begun with the instructors warming us up. They were focusing on the upper ranks, telling them to "Pick it up!" We were then paired up to work our techniques together, such as combinations and kenpos. The instructors concentrated on the upper ranks but checked us out. If we were doing well, we were told to move on to the next combination, but if we were not doing the technique correctly, we had to repeat it over and over until it was right.

We got some rest because the upper ranks had more material, but even though we were beginners the adrenaline was pumping and we were focused. It was impossible to tell how long the test lasted, but finally it was over and it was time to sit on the floor with our eyes closed while the instructors reviewed the results. Soon our hearts leapt: Andrea and I had made yellow belt! As we were presented with our certificates and our new belts, the master also passed along words of wisdom. Our school had a reputation for testing well. We worked hard to prepare and it showed.

One day Master Inman wanted the yellow belts to work on their low stances and had us go into the back room and line up. He pulled out some concrete slabs and told us to put out our arms. Not sure if he was kidding, we did so, getting as low as we could—then he placed the slabs on our arms. I thought my knees would go out any minute, but they were holding up. Master Inman had us deep breathe and focus on something. After about two minutes he could see that we had had enough. He had accomplished his purpose: our stances were lower and we were focusing. It was a good lesson: to focus on the present, forgetting the past or the future. It really did help us to stand more weight for a period of time—otherwise we would all have broken toes!

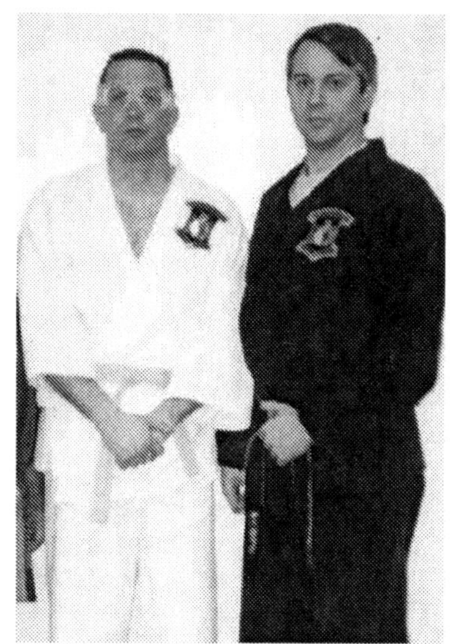

Shawn at Yellow Belt, with Master Kevin Inman

10

Moving Up

Cream always rises to the top.

Sensei Peter Jordan

Starting work on my next rank, orange belt, it was soon evident that each rank became progressively more difficult, but I was getting stronger and my breathing was easier. My focus was improving, with less talk and more action. Master Inman had us constantly refining and improving our kicks, strikes, blocks and other material. Each test was longer and more intense than the last. We had a reputation as a tough school and making it through the ranks was no picnic. Through the discipline and hard workouts I had developed a lot of respect for those who had gone before me.

Andrea and I had moved up to the front row in the class, traditionally reserved for the higher ranks. The beginner class only included the first three ranks: white, yellow and orange belt. When we had earned our purple belts and exchanged our white *gis* for black, we would advance to intermediate class and return to the back row.

I was one of the lucky ones, as I had Andrea to keep me focused and help me practice. My techniques, however, were always a little different from the rest of the students. Master Inman adapted many of them, but now I could adapt them for myself by seeing others perform them. By drilling and drilling, by attending class three or four times a week and taking private lessons, I was able to keep up with the material and the rest of the class. It was difficult, as I had work and school also on my mind but somehow I always found a way to do it. Andrea was a tremendous help in working out with me at home. Most people didn't think we would make it to black belt before killing each other, but we respected each other's efforts and we both wanted it!

Practicing for purple belt brought the intensity level up even more, and to add to the stress of the test, there would be students from another school present along with their instructors, all of whom were new to us. Again, we were faced with blank expressions and tested with new situations.

After the test, one of the instructors from another school came over and introduced himself to Andrea and me. Chris Keith, Sensei, congratulated us on a tough test well done, which made us feel very good. He had been one of the most intense instructors there, but was very pleasant afterwards. It was a great day for us.

We were faced with yet another new situation when we tested for our blue belts on September 19, 1995—just over a year since we had started with Masters of Self-Defense. The test was going to be held in another school in Kennebunk and would have students from three schools. There would also be advanced rank testing.

That night would turn out to be one we would never forget. We had heard that Master Inman was not in a good mood and the Dojo was much smaller than the one we were used to. The instructors, as usual, put on their emotionless faces and showed no expression or familiarity with any of their students. The basics were long and hard and felt as if they would never end, and then we went on to techniques. Students were getting thrown here and there and we had to keep aware so we would not trip over them. The test seemed to go on all night, pushing us to the edge of our limits both physically and mentally, but finally it was over. Again we met Sensei Keith, this time in the rainy parking lot, and he congratulated us on a great job. It meant a lot to me to have Chris Keith Sensei's praise. He was always tough, but I got the sense that he just wanted me to do my best. Anything less was unacceptable.

Now that we were out of the beginner ranks the classes were even tougher, and Andrea and I were more absorbed in the martial arts, reading books and watching martial arts movies from a different perspective. We attended tournaments and took as many classes as we could, including the Tuesday sparring class. At first we did sparring drills to the air, finally getting to use all our kicks and punches, then worked circuit training, going from one station to the next. I built up strength, speed and agility, but my instructor said I needed to be lighter on my feet. Having always preferred a rooted stance with fast striking and countering, I told the master that I was slow on my feet and could not catch the other students. He advised me to let them come to me instead and taught me to prevent my opponent from getting in on me by cutting him off, giving me time to use my strong right arm and foot for quick strikes. After a few months of sparring, the other students started to respect what I could do and were not as quick to count me an easy win after getting trapped on the inside with my strength and speed.

I took my licks, however. There was a lot of trial and error learning what my strong points were, then learning to use them to my advantage. When we sparred with advanced ranks, they would work their evading skills as they knew better than to get in the range of my strikes. I always fell for the fakes until the master taught me how to look at body movement to see where my opponent would dodge. He would let me make mistakes and then helped me to figure out the correct response to each new situation.

As you advance beyond beginner ranks, you are expected to start learning weapons. I remember the day I had my first sword lesson. It was a katana or Samurai sword and although I was really excited about playing with it, it was not at all what I had expected. You need extreme focus and concentration to handle a sword without cutting your leg off. Master Inman started me off with a practice sword that weighed the same as the real thing but was not sharp—thank goodness, or I would be missing several body parts! While practicing striking, I hit my leg several times, which hurt but at least it didn't cut. After weeks of practice I finally improved my focus and concentration to the point of not hitting myself, at which point Master Inman said I was serious enough to try the sharp sword . . . though I noticed that he moved to the farthest side of the room just in case. I reminded him that he had told me I had improved, but he smiled and said, "Not that much."

One day I came into the Dojo and there were many poles set up in a circle, each with a lit candle upon it. Master Inman was attempting to cut off each wick with the sword and put out the flames. I knew he was practicing, so, figuring that this was going to be good, I sat down quietly to watch. He put out a few candles on his first attempt; the second time he hit two of them, knocking them down. After waiting for what seemed like an eternity, I stood up and walked over to him. He said he hadn't realized I was there and I told him I didn't want to break his concentration.

"I'm only practicing—getting ready for a demonstration for a tournament." I wanted to say something about his need for a lot more practice but did not want to seem disrespectful. To be honest, I thought he was terrible but did not want to hurt his feelings.

The next week the whole school went to the tournament to see Master Inman's demonstration. The whole place was packed and buzzing with anticipation—but I was the exception. I was apprehensive after what I had seen in practice. Master Inman came out with his sword, and in the blink of an eye took out every wick in the circle of candles. But it was not over! My instructors were holding up fruit, watermelons and cantaloupes. He picked up two razor-sharp kamas and in mere seconds, fruit slices were flying through the air. Then several brown belts attacked him with Bo's and he handled them easily. The last demonstration was one of focus and concentration. He stretched out between two chairs; head on one and feet on the other while several concrete slabs were placed on his midsection, then students with sledge hammers broke them. It was a terrific demonstration!

The following week I asked Master Inman how he had gotten so good in just one week. He told me that he had heard me come in and played being clumsy to fool me. I always looked at things differently from that point on. It's all in the interpretation of what you see.

I enjoyed coming in early to talk with him. He had a great passion for the arts and I was always looking for new knowledge. We talked about Zen philosophy among other subjects and played the game of asking each other Zen questions such as "Is the glass half empty or half full?" I learned how to look at life situations differently as well as how to deal with them as they happened and enjoyed his martial arts stories, especially the ones where he didn't do all that well. I realized that most martial artists were not born skilled; they all went through what every student who aspires to a black belt goes through. The instructors at our school were all very good. Many of them are still our friends today and are still teaching.

Purple belt to blue belt: intermediate ranks. Drilling harder, kicking and punching longer. More sit-ups and stretches-this was a different class than the beginners'; much more intense. I had better stamina and was getting more muscular; more rooted, focused, concentrated. On Saturdays we had a class that included all adult students from beginner white belt to black belt. Warm-ups were done by the whole class and then we broke up into beginner, intermediate and advanced. Each martial arts style and system has its own, particular belt colors, but they all start with a white belt and end with black.

Sensei Dustin Boyington comments: I first met Shawn when I was an orange belt training in Master Inman's Dojo. Shawn was just starting and I was very concerned for him, as Master Inman was notoriously hard on students. He showed them no favors. I was certain that Shawn would give up after a few weeks, but I was so wrong! We came up in the ranks together. Although I was always at least one rank ahead of Shawn, he pushed me to the limit, showing me how spirit and discipline motivated him to exceed his potential and could motivate me also.

Everyone accepts Shawn and marvels at him: his ruggedness, his spirit; his energy. Shawn wants to know everything; wants to learn and eats up any and every instruction he can get, not only in Kenpo Karate, but in Jujitsu, Chi Kung, Wing Chung, Chi-Na, Tai Chi and in every weapon he can lay his hands on! He constantly challenges me to do better.

I had to learn everything the way the class worked it and then I had to figure out then learn the adaptations. This would be a great help to me later as an instructor for the physically challenged; it was hard to keep up with the class but I loved martial arts, even though my body was taking a beating but, every day I was getting closer to a black belt. My work at the hospital was going well and I was promoted to cardiac stress technician performing patient stress-testing and heart monitoring. I was still working full-time and attending college part-time. My math skills were rusty, having been out of school a long time and I had to have tutoring, but everything was going well.

Christopher Keith
Sensei, 5th dan

During the fall of 1994 I owned and operated a martial arts school in North Windham, Maine. This school was part of the Masters system, a group of New England Kenpo schools. On a warm, sunny Saturday, several students from my school traveled to Portland where they would be tested for new belt ranks together with students of Master Kevin Inman in the Portland Masters school.

They were going for beginner ranks of yellow and orange, and intermediate ranks of purple and blue. The atmosphere in the Dojo was charged, with two dozen students about to put their abilities on the line. My students were excited to be part of a test taking place on the floor of a larger, out-of-town Dojo. As I then held the rank of sandan, 3rd degree black belt, I had applied three red velour stripes to my black belt that stood out against my black gi. I did it for effect; as I owned a school and worked night and day as chief instructor; small things such as stripes and awards add to the impression. (Today, I only wear a plain black belt, even when administering a black belt test.)

One new process we had in store for the candidates was requiring them to perform basics and follow some commands solo-out in front of the group. Performing in isolation put a little more pressure on each one. I could see shades of disappointment creep across some faces as the students retired from the firing-line knowing that they had blown one or two commands.

Master Inman at godan or 5rd degree was the testing master. At one point, he gave me the floor and I ran the students through kenpos or self-defense techniques in a group. I maintained a stern demeanor as I shouted out the numbers, kiais, types of attacks and the like. When a student froze and failed to react, they were made to do pushups immediately. Nothing slipped past unobserved. The early afternoon light came through the lobby past the front office, as well as through the doors at the back of the Dojo that had been left open to let in light and air. The students were striving and their sweat was proof. Understand: the test was designed to get the students to succeed. Being tough on them just made them happier: the tougher the test, the tougher they felt they were!

Towards the end of the test, the candidates again came out solo to perform katas and pinans, which are movements usually about one minute long that demonstrate typical fighting moves in the karate style. One orange belt came out and took a little longer to perform his pinon. The student was Shawn Withers. His body was thin and noticeably asymmetrical. His movements were halting, and it was apparent that he had not been capable of athletic endeavor for some time. He could hardly step forward. The range of his blocks and strikes was restricted. I lost track of the time he was taking to perform his pinon. Time no longer mattered. What mattered and what transfixed me as well as everyone else in the room was Shawn's determination to face this moment and carve out that kata as best as he possibly could. As if the stepping forward moves were not enough, the pinon contained pivots to the rear which Shawn somehow managed. I asked myself why he had picked a physical therapy so difficult. At last he finished. The normal passage of time resumed.

I met Shawn in the lobby after the test. He was with a pleasant lady who had also tested, and I learned she was his wife, Andrea. I was glad for both of them. Students came out of the shower and locker areas. Their mood was one of relief; thrilled that the test was over and hopeful that more progress was ahead. Talking with my students later that Saturday, I found that their focus was on one student only: the student whose performance had floored everyone-Shawn Withers. The courage, nerve and sheer guts in Shawn's performance humbled us. We all doubted that, had we faced a similar physical obstacle, we would be capable of getting out there; trying to hang on and pushing the way he had to get the job done.

The following year on a rainy night in Kennebunk, the instructors and selected students from four Masters schools gathered for a test at Bill Allaire's Dojo on Route 1. Shawn was present wearing-I believe-a purple belt. The room was packed with martial artists and the front windows were black and streaked with raindrops. At least seven black belts attended to vouch for their students as well as to administer the test. Under Master Inman's command, the black belts drove the students through their self-defense drills in a fury. As the evening took shape, the

Master's mood soured. It seemed to me he was dissatisfied with the level of effort of some of the students. His dissatisfaction mounted. Candidates performed the same maneuvers over and over again, and in the process they tired so that individual performances gradually deteriorated. The black belts took seats in front of the students, all remaining silent as the master lectured. Heads hung in disappointment at their inability to deliver what we all prized: the flow of high skill, high effort and success. Even the best among them were stung by the Master's criticism.

"This can take all night if it has to. The black belts here don't have to be anywhere. It can take as long as you want."

Their sweat cooled on them dangerously. Some, I know, questioned why they had ever become involved with these instructors and why they had ever believed in this system. In time-mercifully-the test ended and promotions were given.

Following the post-test briefing from the master, and after congratulating my students, I was happy to get out in the fresh air of the parking lot. I put my gym bag in the trunk of my car and closed the trunk. I looked back at the entrance to the Dojo across the rainy parking lot and saw Shawn and Andrea coming out carrying their gear. I walked across to them to congratulate them on their promotions. I hadn't seen either of them since the beginner level belt test the previous summer. Both were remarkably improved. None of us mentioned the brutality and frustration of the test that had just taken place.

In those days, I only saw Shawn sporadically as I did not train in the same Dojo. Years later, Shawn told me that he had never forgotten the fact that I had walked back across the parking lot in the rain to congratulate him. I guess you never know exactly how much an action of yours will affect another person.

Several years have passed and Shawn and Andrea Withers have both attained nidan, or second-degree black belt in Northern Chi Martial Arts, our kenpo system. At their second-degree test, I witnessed incredibly worthy performances by true fighters. The bulk of Shawn's body was powerful; his momentum unwavering. His broad, rounded back and his signature blows made me name him the Bearcat. I called him the Bearcat because he had developed his own way; his own style of fighting, of deporting himself. He had his own system, his own techniques, some of which he called 'one-armed.' He had come into his own-he had reached the goal and found himself in the martial arts.

I have never before-or since-witnessed the quality or the extent of the physical transformation in a person through martial arts or any other therapy that I have observed in Shawn.

Over the past few years, Shawn has attended many classes with me in Tai Chi and Chi Kung. One winter session, he and a lady were the only students. We spent many challenging and gratifying hours together and-because of his assiduous study and his work with people who are physically challenged-I now consider Shawn to be a fellow instructor of Chi Kung.

Cardiac Trouble

When you come to the edge
of all the light you have known
and are about to step out into darkness . . . .
Faith is knowing one of two things will happen ...
there will be something to stand on
or you will be taught how to fly.

Anonymous

In November of 1995 we were getting ready to test for blue belt when everything came to a halt. In the previous May, I had been at my brother's house, playing football with my nephew, Wayne. Suddenly, I was completely drained of all strength and was winded and sweating far more than I did normally. The football felt as if it weighed 100 pounds. I felt a little dizzy, but I didn't want to scare Wayne or panic him, so I just told him I needed a break; I was getting old. I knew it wasn't that because I usually outlasted the kids and I didn't want to alarm anyone, so I convinced myself that it would just go away with rest.

Andrea was not very comfortable with my explanation when I arrived home. She questioned me and I agreed to go to the emergency room to be checked out. It wasn't difficult to get seen immediately with my cardiac history. My cardiologist was not there that weekend, but Dr. Paul Sweeney was covering. He reviewed my information and came back in the room with a rather unpleasant look on his face and seemed angry. He told us that my aortic valve was small and I was trying to pass blood through it too fast-as if I was trying to pass a gallon where there was only room for a pint. I was admitted and they did a cardiac catheterization. It showed just what I knew I already had: aortic stenosis with an aortic semilunar valve with two leaves instead of the normal three. The symptoms went away and no surgery was planned although they did have me see a surgeon who specialized in valve surgery. The summer went by uneventfully. Andrea and I went camping and hiking and we tested for our blue belts. I was surprised at how good I felt physically.

However, in the fall I noticed that I was weaker and got tired more easily. After the scare of the spring, I didn't want to take any chances, so I called my cardiologist and got an appointment to see the surgeon.

Patricia Stogsdill, MD writes, "Shawn had Aortic Stenosis and underwent a Ross procedure in 11/95. His pulmonary valve was put into aortic valve position and his pulmonary valve was replaced with a tissue valve. He then developed a left ventricle aneurysm in 7/97 that required surgical repair."

I am the luckiest man to have a wife who always has a way of getting me going-not that she wasn't as concerned as I was. My first open heart surgery didn't go as easily as I thought it would. Confident that I would be up and running around in a week or so, I found myself completely drained. I thought I would never do martial arts again. Andrea returned to class after a month had passed because I asked her to do so and to tell the teachers and our fellow students that they hadn't killed me off that easily and I would be back.

My nephew Wayne was now taking the same classes. He was physically gifted and made every move look easy. Almost two months after my surgery, he was in a Christmas tournament at our school that I attended. I was greeted warmly by everyone, but they all looked as if they were seeing a ghost! I felt fine, but suddenly caught a glimpse of myself in the floor-length mirrors of the Dojo. At first I didn't realize I was looking at myself. That was some scary dude in the mirror-he was just skin and bones! Then I realized that I was seeing myself. That was a rude awakening and was responsible for getting me going again. When I left the tournament, I told everyone that I would be back soon. For the next month or so, I walked a lot and slowly began to exercise at home, attempting to eat more in an effort to get back to my original weight. I practiced with Andrea, who helped me with my memory which was still foggy from the cardiopulmonary bypass machine that I had been on so long. They call it 'Pump head.'

Each week I got stronger. I slowly went back to work, and then to martial arts. I hadn't lost any material because Andrea had kept me updated and I kept getting stronger and more proficient.

Andrea and I were scheduled for our next test about four or five months after my surgery. She could have tested earlier, but we had made a pact that we would only test together. It was decided to give us a private test as the teachers were still worried about my strength and endurance. I never wanted to do that again as it meant that Master Inman watched us very closely. Usually we were tested in large groups where the instructor's attention is divided. Now it was just the two of us. Master Inman had a habit of staring at his students during a test that was quite unnerving. We did make mistakes, but we always got back up and tried again. We passed, but now the true work was just beginning as we were at the highest of the intermediate levels, blue belt with a stripe. Months were flying by. I was back to work, karate and school and hadn't time for much else.

Four months later we were ready to advance again, this time for green belt, and it was going to be a rough test. There were several black belt instructors there and many people testing at the same time. You had to get yourself physically and mentally ready for these tests, knowing they would be long and hard. We were well prepared, having drilled long and hard to get ready. The test went well and I was pumped up as usual with the adrenaline rush that comes with the physical and mental effort that goes into testing. I ended up sparring with one of the best students, a brown belt going for 1st degree brown. He had probably been told to go easy on me, but they didn't tell me so I came charging out of the changing room having completely forgotten to put on my protective gear. I felt a little foolish, but was ready to go. I was told to go hard. That wasn't my problem-my problem was trying to slow down. I sparred hard and fast, not giving my opponent a chance to get much in and the sparring went well. When the test ended shortly after, I was wiped out. We always give our all on these tests and they are both mentally and physically exhausting. The instructor who trained you will take it hard if you haven't given your all, but only you are responsible for your efforts.

Green-with-Stripe-each time it got harder and classes were more intense. It seemed as if they were trying to break us but they were only challenging us to improve the level of our skills, but the harder it became, the more I liked it. After each open heart surgery, I always felt that I had to prove myself to myself again. I was going to classes three or four times a week with an occasional private lesson to get all the modifications I had to have. I practiced at home and also assisted instructing classes when needed.

Master Inman had moved his school to a new location, a tennis and racquetball club. There were two Dojos: one a racquetball court and the other, an upstairs ballroom with chandeliers. I broke one during

Bo practice and the other students thought it was funny. I didn't.

Master Inman was going to retire; I think he wanted to give us one really good last workout for the green-with-a-stripe test. The test was long and hard and he was very particular, paying close attention to hand and foot placement. I sensed frustration in him; it must have been difficult to let go of something that you have been doing for so long. An era in martial arts was ending and it was hard to see it end. 3-31-97, the day I received my green-with-a-stripe belt and the day Master Inman retired, is a date I will never forget.

The chief instructor, Sensei Peter Jordan, took over the school with his partner, Sensei Kate Archeambault. He had been with Master Inman longer than the other black belt instructors and had experience running the school for the master. He had dedicated himself to the school and had the same workout ethic as the master: train, train, hard, harder! I looked on it as a new beginning and a learning experience. It was difficult for Peter and Kate to take over from the master and reorganize. I helped out with classes and began to learn the business side of martial arts. I had some sense of the business from Master Inman as I had told him that I would have my own school someday so he would warn me of things to avoid.

Sensei Peter had a very different philosophy from the Master. Peter would work us just as hard, if not harder, but he would work out with us instead of drill, drill and correct. He was very much a hands-on instructor. He wanted to feel you kick and punch and work your technique against him in order to be sure you were doing it correctly. One day Sensei Peter had me punch in for him. He always told us to punch hard and focused, keeping control or you would be showing disrespect for your partner who would not be able to get the technique right. He looked away for a brief moment and told me to punch. I did so without hesitation and hit hard to the sternum. It made a nasty crack that everyone heard. I was shocked when he didn't block it. His shoulders rounded a little and I waited to get a beating, but he just smiled and told us that it was his fault. Sensei Jordan to this day is on guard when he is training and says he learned a valuable lesson. In turn, I told him that I would never show him disrespect by throwing a slow punch.

Classes were going well and I was learning a great deal as it was getting more difficult as I trained for my brown belt. I still felt great from my heart surgery. I had more private lessons with Sensei Jordan who modified the material as needed. It was a learning process for both of us and we usually came up with a technique that was better than the original. Between home, work, martial arts and school, I was tired, but I was used to digging and finding an extra supply of energy from somewhere.

It was time for the routine visit to my cardiologist and the usual tests. I felt and looked well, but looks can be deceiving. He found something abnormal on one of my tests and after further testing, told me that something had let go and I needed to have further open heart surgery. He admitted me to the hospital. I went from Superman to crumbling mess in a very short time. When you go through surgery, your family goes through it with you. We had survived one operation and had barely gotten over that. Things were going so well with work, school and karate. I was mentally crushed by this news. Andrea is the toughest person I know but this would hurt her and my family. I knew what would be coming-pain, pain and more pain, then a long, slow recovery. The previous experience was brutal and it had felt as if it had nearly killed me. I was in no hurry to feel that again and I wasn't sure that I would agree to more surgery. When I discussed my feelings with Andrea, she told me she would back me up no matter what I decided. But the decision really came down to living or dying quickly. The will to live is strong and built in, and I was scared. The surgery would be scheduled quickly and I wouldn't have to think about it for long. I wanted to go home and the doctor agreed as long as Andrea-my very own cardiac nurse-stayed with me, and the surgery was scheduled for later that week However, the next day I was asked to go in the following day and I bit the bullet and said "Yes."

The surgery went well, or so I was told and I was home in three days. It really helps when your wife is your private nurse. I was away from martial arts about 12 weeks again and became, as before extremely deconditioned. Sensei Jordan came to visit and dropped off a martial arts book. I told him I would be back, but I don't think he believed me, but I recovered faster this time and was stronger with Andrea's help in getting me back in shape while making sure I didn't do too much.

Four months after surgery I was testing for my 3rd degree brown belt. Andrea and I had worked really hard; I had been through hell and back and was tired. A lot had happened to me and I was feeling overwhelmed. I did a lot of reflecting on my martial arts and the journey I had gone through to get to where I was now. I felt like a hamster on one of those little wheels, using a lot of energy but not sure where I was going. I spoke to Sensei Jordan about my frustration and I told him that I wasn't sure if I could continue with martial arts. To my surprise, he told me that he had no intention of holding my hand. It didn't matter to him if I stuck it out or quit. My first impulse was to kick him in the head but I came to my senses and left. He had angered me and now I was fired up- he couldn't kill me off! I came back to class more determined and focused and worked twice as hard. What Peter had said had been just what I needed to climb out of my rut.

The 2nd degree brown belt test was a lot longer and we went through all our material. As usual, my body seemed to fight the test at the beginning basics, then I heated up and was ready for anything that was thrown at me. Peter Jordan always worked us twice as hard as the test required and we were always ready for anything. We were well prepared for the changes in the material that were inevitably thrown in and could think on our feet. It was a great preparation for the black belt test that was in our near future. It was not as exciting to put those little black stripes on the brown belt, but each one brought us closer to black belt.

About one month after the 2nd degree brown test I was at work at the hospital in the cardiology unit on the eighth floor when I began to get a little confused and disoriented around noontime. My supervisor knew me well and, concerned, took me to the ER. He suggested that my blood sugar must be low, but I had never had any problems with hypoglycemia in the past. In the elevator down to the ER I felt myself getting more confused and it made me very nervous as I didn't know what was happening. My supervisor called my wife to join me in the ER. She had worked the night shift in the Special Care Unit and was home asleep. I didn't think there was a problem with my heart as I had just passed a very strenuous cardiac test without any problem. The ER doctor insisted on a head CT scan, even as Andrea was urging him to call my cardiologist. The CT scan just showed the results of my stroke in 1982, but they still wanted a neurological exam because of the confusion. By then, the cardiologist had been called and was on his way. He wanted to do a trans-esophageal echocardiogram in order to get a good picture of my heart and it was scheduled for the next day. Meanwhile, I was to be admitted. The fuzziness was clearing and I was realizing that this was going to be serious.

Getting myself ready for the worst-case scenario, I didn't sleep well that night. I knew what the TEE would be like as I had seen this done many times and had experienced quite a few myself. I had worked with the cardiologist doing the procedure many times and he tried to make light of the test and put me at ease, but I knew that something was wrong. Once again, the aortic valve was in need of repair. I needed open-heart surgery yet once more. I told him that I might not have it, in spite of the consequences. The last surgery had been mentally and physically very stressful and I wasn't sure I had it in me to go through that again. I was told that I was young, had a great life, and would lose everything if I didn't have the valve fixed. My survival instincts kicked in; I love life and my wife too much so I decided to have the surgery although I knew that the odds of coming out without any complications were less each time. I asked the surgeon to double-stitch everything he put in, get plenty of rest that night and make sure his glasses were clean. This was the third time this man would touch my heart and I figured he knew where everything was by now.

My family were all devastated by the news and they came to visit with long faces. I was mentally exhausted and I think my brain had shut down. I tried to put on a happy face and cracked a couple of jokes but everyone knew just how serious my situation was. It seemed strange and surreal and I remember thinking that, if no one left me, the surgery couldn't begin.

Early the next morning I was prepped. As usual, everything was shaved which always gave me a chill. Then came the long, lonely ride on the gurney down to the operating room during which it was hard to stay mentally positive, but saying good-bye to Andrea was even worse. I was put on the table and IVs were hooked up. I was asked to count down from ten, but I just asked them to do a good job and out I went.

I woke up with the usual tubes in place and my body numb from the medications. The endotracheal tube was most bothersome and made me restless but I was so tired. I didn't want to move because of the pain in my chest. My body had gone though hell yet once more. I was told that a very large mechanical valve had been placed in my heart. Andrea and my father were the only visitors allowed before the endotracheal tube came out. It must have been difficult for them to see me in pain and feel helpless. I found it hard to sleep as the constant clicking noise made by the valve was hard to shut out of my consciousness. I was morbidly waiting for it to stop, which would have meant I was in deep trouble!

Tubes were removed one at a time and I felt-and probably looked-more human. I was helped out of bed and began to walk around the room and began to feel that recovery was possible. The nursing staff were excellent. I'm sure that having my wife working on the unit helped, but if I couldn't sleep because of the sound of the valve, someone would come and listen to me.

I was out of the hospital in three days after surgery as there was a bed shortage in the step-down intensive care unit and I did have my own private intensive care nurse at home. I couldn't have gone through a third surgery without my wife's support and her nursing care. She is truly my love, my partner and my best friend.

At home, my only task was to recover and to get back to martial arts, which was a passion by now. Before I could go back to the Dojo there was a minimum of 12 weeks to heal my sternum. I took little steps. I visited the school and watched classes to get me pumped up and began to slowly work through forms and techniques with Andrea at home to keep my memory of them. As I slowly recovered, I went back to work part-time, then full-time. When I started back at karate again everyone was a little nervous about working out with me except Peter. He would try out soft strikes to the sternum to make sure I was OK. I did have restrictions now because I was on anticoagulation therapy. I could work out as hard as I could, but had to avoid a lot of hard contact or getting thrown to the ground. I really appreciate all my fellow students who were my ukes (training partners) and let me take them down. In retrospect, I was a little insane for pushing myself to my limit, but I was getting back into condition and proving to myself that I could survive anything.

Peter Jordan remembers: "When he had to have his first open-heart surgery in 1995 we were very concerned. This was serious surgery and very risky, but Shawn, incredibly, sailed through it. What impressed me more than anything else about Shawn was the fact that, although he had been out for 12 weeks, he started right up exactly where he had stopped! He accomplished this, as he told me, by constantly practicing all his moves in his head, so even if he returned physically weaker he had not forgotten anything. Shortly after, in 1997, he had a tear and had to have a valve repair-more risky open-heart surgery and I was even more worried. He'd survived one; could he make it through two? Again, he made it, and again he started back at the point he had reached before the surgery. Then he had an artificial valve replacement in June of '98 and was back in the hospital with even more open-heart surgery. I couldn't believe that he would survive yet another dangerous operation, but he did, came back, went on to get his black belt and start Like Water.

He is an amazing guy. I have never known anyone like Shawn. He has the most tremendous drive to overcome his disability and succeed in whatever he attempts. He also will do anything for one whom he considers a friend, dropping what he is doing at a moment's notice and coming to you if you need him. I've known him as a student, a fellow instructor, but most of all as a friend and an inspiration to everyone he touches.

13

The Waiting Room

Come what come may,
Time and the hour runs through the roughest
day.

William Shakespeare, Macbeth

Kathi writes:

Friday, June 19, 1998. 7 AM: So begins the wait. No-actually, the wait began the moment we received news that you were in the hospital. We knew, without knowing, it was going to be bad news. You know the rest, but maybe what you don't know is what really goes on in the waiting room. I'm writing this to give you a little insight and-if the truth be known-this is my way of holding it all together.

As I had observed everyone waiting during the last two surgeries, I had thought, "I wish Shawn could actually feel all the love, all the worry and heartache that is taking place in this walled and glassed cubicle here in SCU (Special Care Unit). I bet we share a common thought: if any one of us could switch places with you to spare you any more pain-physical and emotional- we would. And then there's the gamut of 'guilt' thoughts and feelings running through our minds . . . Let's start with me-the way I had lit into you during your last visit at my house-finally speaking my mind-only to the wrong person: my brother, who only wanted to jive over Java . . . and I had to choose to be tough that day. Oh, of course I always rationalize the lack of time we spend together as due to the fact that we all lead full and busy lives but now, as I sit here I realize how empty my life would be without my family . . . my brother. I make promises in trade for prayers and-you know-I've kept a lot of the promises I made here in this very room. I won't bore you with how, but I have kept them because of the sheer gratitude of seeing you after each surgery.

The others in the waiting room too . . . they all have the guilt-knowing you, you must get a chuckle out of this-yeah, they have it too! Maybe it was an argument with you, or perhaps someone knows that they could put more into their relationship with you; whatever the reason, you can see it on their faces. You can almost see them making the 'deal' with God. I bet you made one, too.

7:10 AM: One of us picks up the newspaper and tries to get involved, another paces the hallway; the pages of a magazine get flipped and dropped back on the table.

Watching them wheel you down the hall . . . it becomes real. The insignificant chitchat dies down and everyone seems to break off and enter into their own world-a very singular world even though we are all here together. We all know that we will be waiting for news, piece by piece, milestone to milestone, of the progress you will be making, alone in body far away in another room. It's as if we cannot protect you now . . . only with our love and prayers. We do know more this time. In my opinion-not good. I think that knowing, but not knowing enough, is too scary. We don't understand the terminology and the pros and cons thing; we only know Fate has handed our brother, our son, our uncle, our husband, another blow.

One thing we all agree on is that, if it was any of us, we'd lie on the floor and kick and scream, then run as fast as we could for . . . well, I guess until we could run no more. You, you on the other hand, will face this as you did the other surgeries, like a ram heading into a wall. Yeah-we know-you're more scared, more tired, more discouraged . . . but still, you're you, and we all know you are unmatched in determination.

Shawn, I believe you were put here to teach us something. Dad said to me the other day, "Shawn has had to fight from the moment he was born-he's been fighting ever since." We all know he's right. We also know that you are the one born with all the drive, all the self-discipline, all the friggin' stamina! But, all is not lost for us poor souls sitting here in the waiting room, we learn from you-we really, really do. Isn't that what you hope for? You always want us to strive; we do, each in our own way.

Without sounding sappy, you know you're my hero. I believe you may be everyone's hero.

8:10 AM: Everyone seems to have settled down to something. Jeff and mom are playing Solitaire-Jeff's probably cheating to put a spin on it. Dad's just sitting there staring. Andy's doing her homework, but I watch her face; her eyes more often than not will be staring off into space, too. She's unbelievable, Shawn, she really, really is. She is your match, she has to be the proverbial 'soul mate' for you. I'd love to have what you have. She answers our questions . . . to her they are probably idiotic, but she answers them patiently and simply for us. I haven't quite figured out her . . . mannerisms-her 'faces.' I can't tell when she's protecting us from information for our sakes. She is weeding it out for us . . . hmm . . . I think she's losing patience with these two women next to us. They're loud and somewhat . . . simple. I think they are getting on her nerves.

It's hard to block out the other visitors' stories, their chatter. In the ten minutes the people sitting next to us have been here, it appears that whoever they have in here is doing very well. I imagine our family talking in the same manner in about 12 hours. I know everything will go well, but I feel the dread of what you have ahead of you. Phase II of that strength test, huh? I have just figured out that they-the women to the left-have a relative who is a baby here.

To be perfectly honest, I think what I am most sick over right now is knowing that the first hurdle those surgeons face with you is getting you opened up. We learned about that during your last surgery when the nurse came down to tell Andy that, when they opened up your chest, they couldn't see the inside of your heart (probably because of adhesions-Andrea).   See-ignorance is bliss! I don't know a whole lot about the rest of the surgery to have these very . . . graphic images in my mind. I know there are certain 'landmarks' throughout the surgery. Each one you pass, each one of your victories will be celebrated down here.

11:00 AM: Hurdle number one-and you cleared it beautifully-they opened you up successfully and the nurse, Laurie, sounded so positive. As usual, Shawn . . . a walk in the park!

So, we all breathe.

11:50 AM: Hurdle number 2, Shawn . . . you're off the pump. I wish you could see Andrea's face-I can read these mannerisms-the relief, the joy. All of a sudden, everyone's tired . . . . Relief takes the form of exhaustion.

I wish I could make you understand that I am saying all this not because I'm whining . . .

Jeff, by the way, says to tell you he gave blood today and he didn't whine once . . . . Seriously, we don't mean to make it seem this is all about us; we realize-to as much an extent as possible-what this is about; who it is about. We (all) know what it means for you. Let me just attempt to shed a little light on what it means for us: we want to take your place so you can go on doing what you want to be doing. We want to think you are not in pain, but if you are, we want to take it away. It breaks my heart. All your hard luck and physical setbacks break all our hearts.

We've named you the Iron Man-it's 1:05 and you are back in your room up here. We are surprised-but then we're not, because you are you. Andrea's beaming and she's out the door.

OK, Shawn, I have to take a minute to celebrate yet another hero in our family. I pause here to mention (again) the (not easily forgotten because he won't let us) fact that your brother, Jeff, gave blood today. He had an overwhelming desire to return something to the community . . . . He wanted to give himself . . . he's filling me in as I write . . . the compassionate, generous, handsome (in a crude way), giving all-around jovial kind of guy! (Whoa, glad I could catch all that.) He feels it necessary to be included in the documentary of your ordeal. As he puts it, what's the big deal about you having a little chest work done when he walked down the long, dark corridors of the old part of this hospital . . . cold, steel tables . . . long scary needles and hairy nurses. Jeff's trauma? His wound? He complained about the size of the hole in his arm to the poor lady sitting next to us!

I think I have done justice to all heroism involved. Now, as we visit here, gathered in a whole different light, we can laugh without guilt and-well . . . go back to talking about the pain-in-the-ass you are.

5:45 PM: Everyone has been in to see you except me. I'd like to think you know I'm here and I love you . . . NOT . . . . You love to see me squirm, to feel the blood all drained out of me. I know, I know-now I know how you feel!

14

Black Belt

No athlete is crowned
but in the sweat of his brow.

St. Jerome
from Letter 14

Four months after surgery I was getting ready for my 1st degree brown belt test. Training was hard, but my heart was in peak condition and I felt a strength in my body that had never been there before the surgery. I came to the Dojo every morning to train with Peter. He started me with Chi Kung meditation to help me get through the harsh workout that followed that were over two hours long. Afterwards, we would go to the local Chinese restaurant for lunch and talk about future plans after my black belt test.

On 11-14-98 I tested for my 1st degree brown belt. Andrea and I were the highest ranks present for this test; it was up to us to pull off a great test, and we did. We made some mistakes but we handled them well and moved on, as martial artists do under pressure, ending with kenpo sparring. No pads, no protective equipment. The instructors thought perhaps that we would go easy on each other, but that us not how we did it; we went long and hard-but controlled. The test lasted about three hours and I tested my heart valve that day. It clicked away, sounding like a very fast watch, but I felt fine. I knew then that I could get through a black belt test.

Martial arts is never boring. Once you have reached one goal, it is time to focus on the next, and in our case it was the black belt test. The training was intense. Peter Jordan told us we needed to be able to do one solid hour of kicking and punching, so we practiced and trained: kick, kick, kick, punch, punch, punch. This type of training makes you strong and hard. I believe Andrea and I were very lucky to have been training then because martial arts have changed a great deal over the last few years. We had gone through ranks with traditional instructors who had ingrained respect and discipline into the students. True, many had dropped out, but those who lasted really knew that they had been through an era in martial arts that probably will not occur again, whether it be for better or for worse. I do not believe there is a right or a wrong way to train in the martial arts. Everyone must find their own way. I trained with no special consideration or treatment: either I made it or I didn't. It may seem barbaric, but I learned a lot about myself and I wouldn't have changed anything. It showed me my strengths and weaknesses and brought out the best in me.

Finally the road to black belt was almost finished. One more test. That is what I had been saying to myself for the last five years: one more test! It finally happened at 9 am on June 6, 1999.

This was to be the toughest test yet. We started out with basics. My adrenaline was up, my blood was pumping. Well trained, we knew how far along in the test we were by which set of material we were working on: basics, kenpos, combinations, grab defenses, etc. My partner was going for his second degree and I had asked him before the test began what it would be like. He told me that sometimes I would feel as if I was dying. He wasn't wrong. I had trained so hard to get into the best shape possible and yet, three hours into the test, I was feeling strain and fatigue. At last came weapons, my favorite then finally, forms. It was now difficult to focus because I was pretty well spent, but then I found 'the zone,' a place where one suddenly becomes focused and the energy all comes from deep down inside. After four hours of going as hard as I could, this zone was strangely calming.

The instructor's job is to find our weaknesses and to attempt to break our focus, but this group of martial artists was very strong and tight. We closed ranks and supported and encouraged each other and sent the message that we would finish this test no matter what! We kept going-and we kept smiling.

Then it was time for the demonstrations and we knew that we were at the end. Our waiting families and friends were invited into the Dojo and the 1st degree black belt candidates demonstrated the presentations they had prepared. At this point, we could barely move, but we all finished our presentations and they were some of the best I have ever seen.

It has been five years since that first black belt test and I have witnessed many tests since, but none like that. It was great to be presented with rank, but it was also a letdown, because I knew that an era had come to an end. It would never be like that again.

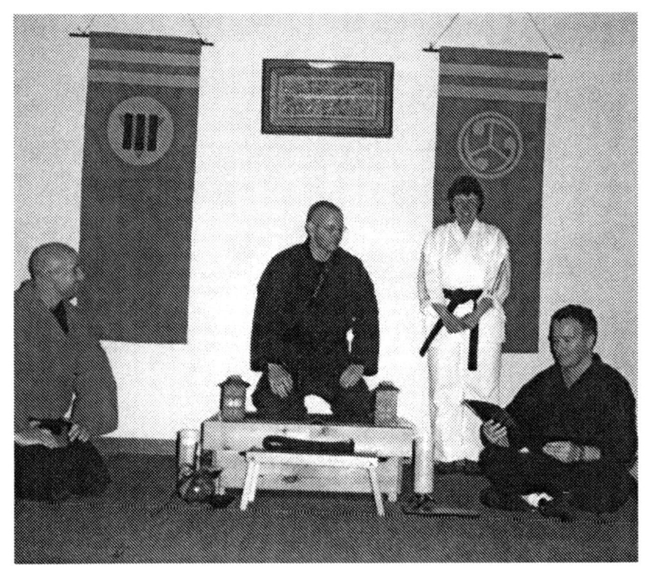

First Degree Black Belt Ceremony

Part III

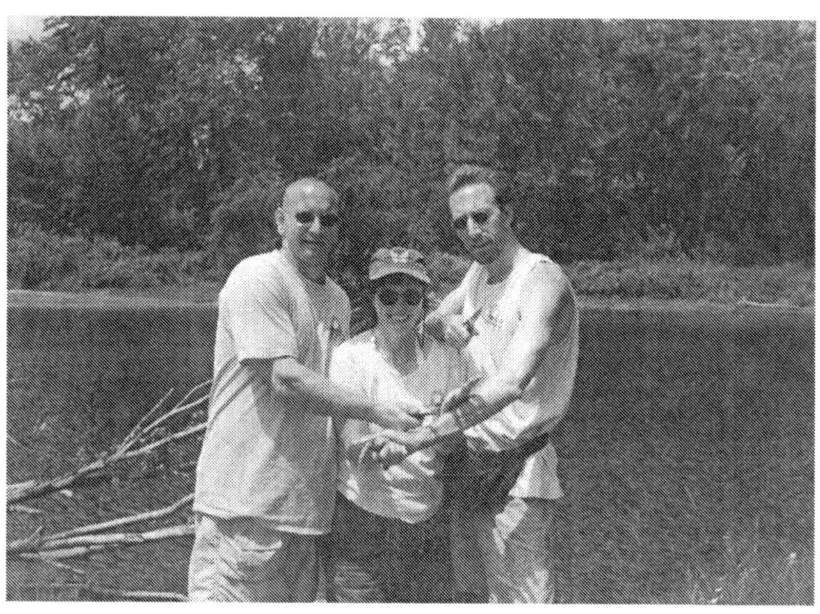

Shawn and Andrea with Doug Young at AMOK! Camp

15

Like Water

> Where your talents and the needs of the world
> cross, there lies your vocation.
>
> *Aristotle*

After the test, we needed a vacation and went camping on Sheepscot Bay. It was early June and there was no-one else in the camp. We had a campsite overlooking the water and it was nice to have the time to just sit back, reflect on what we had accomplished and to speculate on where we were going. We knew that we were barely at the beginning of the journey and many different paths could be explored from where we were. When you are working toward your black belt, you are very focused on the system you are studying, mastering the basics of that system. When you become a black belt, it is as if your eyes now open to the entire world of martial arts. There was so much out there for those who want it that we were like kids in a candy store!

Before I earned my black belt we had been studying the AMOK! system for about two years. It is a style of knife fighting based on Filipino martial arts and was developed by Professor Tom Sotis, truly one of the best knife-fighters in the world. We continued to study AMOK! with Sensei Doug Young in Maine and of course, continued to prepare for our next rank in the kenpo system with Sensei Peter Jordan as well as attending seminars given by many great martial artists such as Dr. Yang Jwing-Ming, Blais Loong, Tony Blauer and CaneMaster Mark Shuey.

When I left Maine Medical Center in October of '98 to attend college full time, I spent a lot of time teaching while I moved up in rank. While I was a green belt, the Aucocisco School-a school for children with learning differences-came to Peter Jordan and asked if they could set up some classes for their students. He asked me to help, thinking that I would be a great role model for these kids. I enjoyed it so much and was so encouraged by the progress the children made, that I told Peter that I'd like to start some classes for people like myself-the physically challenged. He agreed that it would be a great idea, but told me that I had to get my black belt first, in order to have credibility with the students-that a black belt gives you all the authority you didn't and couldn't have the day before you earn it!

While I was working on my black belt, I enrolled in Northern Chi's Portland, Maine Instructors College and was the first brown belt/Sempai certified instructor graduated from there. I studied Kenpo Karate, Tai Chi, Wing Chun, Filipino and Russian martial arts and earned my first degree black belt in June '99 and my second degree in June '01.

Shortly after I got my first degree black belt, Andrea, Peter Jordan, Kate Archambault and I started the Like Water Foundation as a nonprofit corporation to bring martial arts to the physically challenged, leasing Dojo space from Northern Chi in South Portland. We divided the work up between us and assembled a small group of very capable and caring individuals to be our Board of Directors. It was quite a learning experience and we discovered it was tremendously hard work to write grant applications, fund raise, keep up with the mountain of required paperwork, recruit students and teach classes, as well as attempting to fulfill our non-martial arts commitments. I found that I was spending 99% of my time fundraising and networking-without a salary and Andrea discovered that writing grant applications was something she was not equipped to do if she wanted to maintain her sanity as well as her job as a cardiac recovery unit nurse, working 12-hour shifts. Eventually we decided to dissolve Like Water Foundation as a nonprofit entity, and on January 2, 2002, Andrea and I incorporated Natural Motion Martial Arts, Inc. for profit.

We teach our martial arts in the form of several programs, each designed to bring them to a group of people in the way that best suits them and their particular disabilities. The Like Water program is the original program, taught several times a week at our school, which is now located in Scarborough, Maine. We have a diverse group of student, ages ranging from teens to over 70. We started out with seven to ten students at each class, as well as any caregivers who wanted to learn. (Our philosophy is that any caregiver is welcome to take classes free.) At first I took everyone who applied, such as paraplegics, stroke patients, blind, brain-injured, patients with muscle diseases, such as MS and arthritics. Kathy Kroll, a physical therapist at New England Rehabilitation Hospital in Portland referred patients who she thought would benefit from the program and many of our original Like Water students are still with us after 5 years. We rank our students and all our original students are now brown, green or green belt with a stripe and all intend to get their black belts. We have several volunteer instructors from area martial arts programs, as well as guest instructors from time to time, such as Senseis Doug Young and Chris Keith.

The REACH program brings our programs to other facilities, such as the IRIS Network for the blind, and the area rehabilitation hospitals and units for the brain-injured and stroke victims, either as weekly classes or one-time introductory seminars. We also include our self-defense seminars in the REACH program.

As students advance in rank, they are required to learn a weapon, and what more appropriate for the physically challenged than the cane? It is the only weapon that can be carried in plain sight aboard an airplane-and yet it can be lethal in self-defense! The principles of cane-fighting are also easily carried over to knife, sword and stick-fighting. I teach the Cane-Tao program as I have studied the cane with GrandMaster Mark Shuey who had started his own system. He was brought in to teach a seminar at a local Dojo for which I am grateful. I think Master

Shuey might be pleasantly surprised that I handle the cane so well with one hand!

GrandMaster Mark Shuey, Sr., Owner of Cane Masters and Founder CMIA says:

I met Shawn at a seminar in Maine with James Bouchard at his school Northern Chi. Shawn came up to me and introduced himself, we talked, and became friends. Right away, I was impressed with his positive attitude and wonderful personality. Over the years, he has constantly shown his desire to help others, never complains about anything, and is always looking for the "good" in life. Shawn has been one of my students since the time we met. He went through the requirements to become a Canemaster, passed with flying colors, and has adapted to teaching others despite his partial paralysis. Shawn has a "never give up" attitude, as well as doing his best to help others where ever he goes. If the world had more people like Shawn, it would be a much better place! I feel proud and privileged that he is one of my Canemasters, and a good friend!

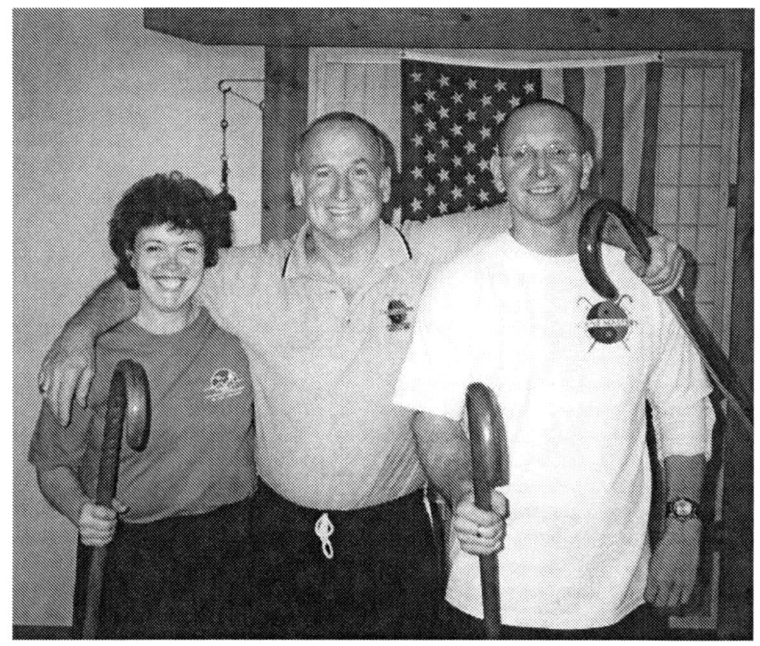

Andrea and Shawn with Grandmaster Mark Shuey, Sr.

I studied and trained with Sensei Dustin Boyington, my loyal friend and dependable training partner who had also attended a seminar with Master Shuey. Dustin helped me work through a lot of techniques and opened my eyes to new material while testing each other to the limit as usual. Ten years younger, he has become the little brother I never had and I have enjoyed training with him for over a decade and continue to do so. He incorporated some Filipino material into our material and then we started to teach students the cane.

We are currently putting together an entire curriculum for cane in manual form for instructors and students.

Dustin comments:

Shawn and I have our differences. For instance: Shawn hates the term 'to flow.' I love it! I am always urging students to flow. I am indifferent to ranks; Shawn thinks that they are extremely important as an incentive for students to strive for; to learn and practice, practice! But no matter what our differences, I consider him my brother. He is closer to me than many of my family are and whatsoever he may need, I will always strive to give it to him.

THE MOONLIGHT WARRIOR

In the darkness of the moonlight
I see a single hand move.
A foot step
A body float.
It then disappears . . . .

. . . . the motion returns.
A movement cuts through the darkness,
First high,
Then low.

Its body shifts, then lunges.
It moves with the cunning of a leopard,
The accuracy of a snake,
Silence of a tiger, balance of a crane
And the spirit of a dragon.

The night masks its skill . . . A well-trained Shaolin.

Who is this warrior? It matters not.

But this one I know as my Sensei, friend and brother . . .
Shawn Withers.

With respect
Dustin Boyington (July 10, 2001)

Douglas James Young, Founder: O-Ki Defensive Arts, Cofounder and Head Instructor: Defensive Tactics Options writes:

I first met Shawn when I gave a seminar at the Portland Northern Chi Martial Arts Center. I was the first time that I had been to their Portland location.

After being introduced by the head instructor I grabbed a student to help with the demonstration of the techniques I was to teach. I had the habit of picking the biggest or toughest-looking guy in the class to do my demonstrations with because, if I use a smaller person, some students might get the idea that the technique will not work against somebody bigger or stronger than I am. That day, Shawn was the one chosen. He looked tough physically and I was to find out after getting to know him that he also has an inner strength to match his exceptional physical martial arts abilities. I'm always sure to tell the person I pick that it is a compliment because, when I pick somebody, I don't want them to get the idea that I'm 'picking' on them. Shawn literally rolled with the punches for a couple of hours and learned the techniques quickly.

I tell people that Shawn is not challenged, but rather that he challenges. I say this because when he is in a class I'm teaching, I always have to come up with a one-handed version of the technique that everyone else is learning-and I usually have to come up with it on the spot. Teaching Shawn has made me a better martial artist and a better instructor.

One of my fondest memories of Shawn is the occasion when I had the honor of presenting him with the International Blade Fighters Guild special Courage Award on behalf of our edged weapons instructor Tom Sotis. I made the presentation at the Northern Chi Christmas party in front of Shawn's fellow martial artists, telling them that the significance of any award is based upon the individual or group giving it. Tom Sotis is one of the most skilled hard-core martial artists in the world and the 'real deal.' He trains some of the world's most elite military, law enforcement and private security personnel. When Tom Sotis uses the word 'courage,' it means something.

Professor Tom Sotis, Founder of AMOK!:

Shawn and I first met when he came to one of my seminars in 1998. His friendly smile and unassuming manner belie his focus and intensity. Shawn is rather outgoing and asked me many questions. Over the years he and his wife Andrea have become close friends of mine.

I have known some handicapped students, but none as dedicated as Shawn. I had no reservations about his potential. Experienced instructors notice that physically talented people are often easily dissuaded when the hard work comes-and it always does-and those who learn at an average or slower rate who are used to laboring for their skills are not so easily discouraged. Even more so for Shawn. Because he has to work harder to negotiate life in general, his spirit has been challenged and mastered in more difficult areas than the practice of martial arts. He is used to hard work; Shawn is a Warrior and I am always proud of the fine example he sets for other Warriors. I fully encourage and endorse Shawn's instructorship believing that he will positively impact every student who studies with him

In 2004 we invited Doug to teach a class at our school as we want to give our students a well-rounded education in the martial arts and it is good for them to be exposed to other perspectives and styles. Andrea and I were pleasantly surprised when Doug took this opportunity to present us with our black belts in his system and we were given special instructor's certificates to teach his O-Ki-Tao Defense System. It was truly one of the greatest honors we have had in our career as martial artists and humbling coming from Doug who is the best combat trainer.

16

Student and Teacher Stories

Experienced instructors notice
that physically talented people
are often easily dissuaded
when the hard work comes . . .
and those who learn at an average or slower rate
who are used to laboring for their skills
are not so easily discouraged.

Tom Sotis

Student Stories

LYNWOOD BILLINGS

I had a massive stroke in 1997 that paralyzed my right side. I was in the hospital for two months and in New England Rehabilitation Hospital for one month, with outpatient therapy after.

I heard about the Like Water program from my therapist at NERH and started the program in

January of 2000. It has been wonderful for me, helping me immeasurably, developing self-confidence and improve my physical as well as my mental condition. I now drive and have married. I think that Shawn is so good at what he is doing for us. He has done more than any other rehab.

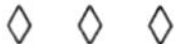

MICHAEL SCHACK

I had a stroke in February 1999 that paralyzed me on my left side, leaving me with a nasty left-sided neglect as well as a nasty attitude. I spent 10 days in MMC and 3 months at NERHP as an inpatient, then almost a year in the out-patient neuro day program.

I met Shawn after being talked into attending a session of Like Water by my recreation therapist Kathy Kroll. Although I was able to walk at that time, my balance was poor and I was easily confused. I remember walking up the steps to the Dojo, tripping halfway up and taking a fall down a few steps.

Like Water has clearly helped me physically regarding strength and balance. Shawn himself was a much larger and more complex form of assistance. First, it was his positiveness and his clear understanding of friendship. It was easy to pick up energy off his drive.

◊ ◊ ◊

ROBERT 'RED' MARSDEN (9-9-44 TO 10-27-02)

There is a very special punching bag in the Dojo, the type known to the martial arts world as 'Bob.' An armless torso of a well-built man with a grim frown on his face, formed out of a hard rubbery substance on an adjustable, water-filled base, it is used for punching, kicking and cane training. Surprisingly, there is a bronzed plaque attached to the base that reads, In memory of Bob 'Red' Marsden-a true Martial Artist. Bob would have loved his memorial and would have been pleased that future martial artists as physically challenged as he was, would use it.

His dear friend and significant other Sonya Mulkern writes about him:

> *Bob had a severe stroke that affected his right side. He was not able to do much until he came to Shawn's program. He improved physically and mentally and was totally inspired by Shawn's ability to overcome any adversity in his life. They were the best of friends. Bob hung all the pictures of the different stages of his development in the martial arts on his walls. All Shawn's students have this pride in their accomplishments. Shawn was a wonderful Sensei*

and friend to both Bob and me and participated in Bob's memorial service.

His classmates remember Bob as a charming, determined and focused, hard-hitting member of the class who, in the last year of his life when he was struggling with so many ailments, still tried to come to as many classes as he could. He and I had a special relationship. Bob was a lifelong Boston Red Sox and New England Patriots fan-both then hapless, losing-at-the-last-minute teams. I bet Bob $10.00 in 2001 that Boston would, as usual, lose this year. When they lost the pennant race at the last minute, Bob paid up graciously, and he wrote a note that, together with the $10 bill, I framed and hung in my office. But Bob got his revenge early the next year, when-to everyone's amazement-the Patriots won the Super bowl and this time, I had to pay up! Bob, you would be amazed to learn-or perhaps you know-that they did it again in 2004, but we all hope that, wherever you are, you are watching all New England celebrating the Boston Red Sox finally winning the World series on October 27, 2004!

Kathy Kroll, a recreational therapist at New England Rehabilitation Hospital had asked me to speak to Bob Marsden about my Like Water program. The memory that remains with me at all times is the sparkle in Bob's eyes-an internal energy waiting to grow.

I was a little concerned when Bob started Like Water. He looked frail and badly in need of exercise. However, I soon learned that Bob came with great determination. No matter what I threw at him, he did it with a smile. He told me he loved karate and it showed by the effort he made in every class. Rain, snow, sleet-Bob would show up early and we would talk. We enjoyed our conversations and developed a great friendship. He always told me a joke before class, but when it got underway he became very serious, had great focus and forgot about the world outside for a couple of hours. He was so very tough on himself but was proud of his accomplishments, which he knew took the discipline, respect, effort that was expected of everyone, regardless of age or ability. He set aside his physical challenges to concentrate on improving himself. He knew he earned his ranks: we did not give them away. We expected everyone to do the same, to go beyond yourself to find your true self within.

He had a great passion for baseball and he loved his company's softball team and managed it.

Bob had multiple health problems towards the end of his life and when he died, his sister asked me to be one of the speakers at the funeral service. It was a privilege and an honor to do so. I was also glad to see most of his fellow students there to honor and remember him.

◊   ◊   ◊

MARIE 'PEGGY' AND MAURICE 'MOE' TOURIGNY

Maurice 'Moe' Tourigny is a silver-haired sweet-faced older man with a perpetual smile-and a grip of steel and two iron fists; his wife Marie (known as Peggy to her friends and fellow caregivers) straight, slender is the rock upon which Moe's life rests. Among Shawn's many student/caregiver teams, theirs is probably the most remarkable story of indomitable courage against incredible odds.

Moe has a history of ill health that commenced from the two heart attacks he suffered at the age of 34, disabling him for seven years. He and Marie had two small children and no income apart from some apartment rentals and a camp they had bought as an investment. Moe received SSDI, which Marie says was peanuts back in 1969. Even though Moe had recovered enough after seven years to take on some of the responsibilities of supervising the rental business that Marie had built up, he still never enjoyed really good health and life was a struggle for them both.

In 1994 he suffered a bleed in his brain that resulted in a clot that resembled-according to the surgeon-a 1/4" thick pancake. He underwent one craniotomy to remove it, after which he suffered an inter cranial hemorrhage. During the second craniotomy two days later to clip the aneurysm he suffered a massive stroke that left him comatose. Marie was told that he would never regain brain function and he would remain in essentially a comatose state. She was urged to give her permission to take him off life support but-a devout Roman Catholic-she refused. Never leaving his side in the hospital for the 44 days he remained there, she prayed for a miracle. There were no doctors in that hospital that ever gave Marie any encouragement and she was told that Moe had only brain stem function.

On the 45th day, he was taken to New England Rehabilitation Hospital, still in a vegetative state. For the first three or four days, Marie stayed by his side, but then consented to go home at night to rest and deal with her sadly neglected business. Moe was at last showing signs of recovering some consciousness that was rather like a very new baby 's growing awareness in his big man's body.

Moe was 55 days in rehab, then was discharged to home. He could barely walk, talk, feed or dress himself. Without any training, without help, all the assistance Marie had was from their son Richard who diligently helped her rehabilitate his dad while juggling his own work schedule. Marie drove Moe back and forth to NERH for the next year to the day program where the therapists worked with him intensively, concentrating on all phases of his recovery. Gradually, he relearned speech-to talk more fluently, to walk more steadily and to regain normal thought processes. By the winter of 2000 he had come a long way mentally but physically was still taking baby steps. For instance, when he needed to change direction in a standing position, he did it just as a toddler would, turning around with many tiny baby steps.

Even though Moe is an avid newspaper reader and takes every newspaper available in the Greater Portland area, Peggy rarely reads them, but one day she just happened to glance at the January 14, 2000, South Portland Sentry. A picture of a young man caught her eye and she read the accompanying headline about a new program that helped people with disabilities learn the martial arts. The program was Like Water, and the young man, Shawn Withers.

Intrigued by the headline and what she says was the love and the kindness she saw in the man's face, she sat down and read the accompanying article, thinking of Moe and his lack of physical ability and self-esteem. Reading about Shawn's recovery from his devastating stroke with his desire to give back what he had learned, she knew that here was something that could help Moe get some of his abilities back. After consulting Maurice, she made the call.

In January of 2000, Moe started classes at Like Water. He has been going every week without fail with the exception of time out for open heart surgery in 2001 and various other ailments. He has progressed from his white gi with a white belt, to a black gi with a green belt, proud to call himself a martial artist, and has his eye set on a black belt. His sparring partners are all too familiar with his steel grip and his iron fists, and also his gentle smile as he delights in his ability to block and strike.

Marie cannot say enough about Shawn and what he has done for Maurice-and for herself.

"I loved the eye contact Shawn made right from the start. His deep sincerity and his dedication to his art and his students shines through. He cares, he loves, he wants and needs to help. Shawn has a God-given gift for teaching the physically challenged."

◊ ◊ ◊

RON FECTEAU/HELEN FECTEAU

Ron, a tall, balding man wearing a brace on his right leg, walks with a cane and his right leg is visibly weaker than his left. He has been with Like Water for three years and was referred by NERH 6 months after a left-sided stroke he suffered in April of 2001. He also had a brain tumor removed when he was 35 years old with subsequent radiation and chemotherapy. He says that Like Water has improved his balance remarkably. Shawn is "a remarkable man and I am still learning."

His wife, Helen, a woman whose tired face and watchful focus on her husband as he struggles to balance through a move is typical of the caregivers at Like Water, is much more informative.

"I'm so happy that Ron has a positive attitude about something and is attempting to get better, to try something new, to look forward to coming to class each week."

She didn't believe him when he came home from NERH 6 months after the stroke and told her that he was starting karate lessons at Like Water and was next Friday OK? She asked him if this was something he wanted to do and he was enthusiastic. So she rearranged her work schedule so that she could drive him and they have been coming every Friday since he started in 2001.

"Like Water has been so good for Ron. He knows that he won't be asked to do anything that is beyond his abilities, but to find out just what he is capable of doing has given him a positive attitude. It is also so good for him to meet others whose strokes were even worse than his as well those who are better and to see what they have achieved at Like Water. He looks forward to coming each week."

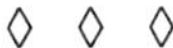

DONNY HEATH

Donny is a twenty-year-old with remarkable, well-groomed dark red hair of which he is very proud, plus multiple disabilities including bilateral hip replacements, a brain cyst and a rod in his back to straighten his spine. His speech is slow and deliberate but with hesitations as he searches for the right word.

"I began to study Shotokan Karate at the age of six and was at green belt level when I had multiple surgeries at the age of thirteen that incapacitated me and instead of karate, I had to start on a long program of physical therapy."

He heard of Like Water at New England Rehab Hospital at the age of nineteen and brings his youthful eagerness and enthusiasm to each class. Even though Shawn teaches Kenpo Karate, it is similar enough to Shotokan that he was able to start Donny off at green belt level with adaptations for his multiple conditions. He quickly relearned all that he needed at this level and soon tested for his next belt-green with stripe and is currently working on his brown belt.

"Shawn has helped me so much with gaining back my strength. I think he is a great martial artist and a great person."

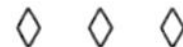

SUSAN LEACH

Furry Slippers

Samisen music and incense float through the Dojo; candles are lit upon a low table in front of the big Stars and Stripes hung upon the far wall. The Like Water class is lined up in front position. Susan Leach is glowing with pride as she bows and receives her green belt in a short, solemn ceremony from Sensei Shawn and Sensei Andrea Withers. Shawn reminds Susan and the rest of the class that no longer is she just a student; she is now recognized as a Martial Artist.

At the celebration after the class, Shawn teases Susan. "Remember when you started with Like Water almost four years ago? You were so unstable that you couldn't walk backwards without falling over-you had to wear your furry L.L.Bean bedroom slippers to keep your balance!" She laughs, but has tears in her eyes as she remembers.

Susan, a short, stocky blonde woman nearing her sixtieth birthday, had been diagnosed with both Multiple Sclerosis and Type II diabetes 18 years previously, not long after she had fallen down a flight of icy stairs and shattered her left ankle so badly that it took four surgeries to repair, ending in fusion and a permanent limp. Coupled with the on-again and off-again coordination and balance difficulties of MS, this earned her a disabled status. She could have just sat back and existed on a lifetime of SSDI but, like Shawn, determined that her life was not yet over, she resumed her career as a Mental Health specialist with the state of Maine, as well as working as a residential counselor and attending UMA part-time to study for a degree in her chosen field.

In January 2000, she read a story in the Portland Press Herald featuring Shawn Withers, his remarkable history and the startup of a new Martial Arts Program for the Physically Challenged-Like Water. All too aware of her tendency to gain weight, she had never dared to attempt any exercise program as she was so self-conscious about her lack of coordination and her ungainly gait, but this seemed to be just for people who were handicapped as she was, and who perhaps would not laugh at her clumsiness. Her life partner, Sylvia, concerned about Susan's physical unfitness, urged her to try the class, and offered to go with her for support whenever she had a Friday off from her evening shift as a nurse. The Dojo was just around the corner from Susan's workplace and, as she too worked the evening shift, she could just make the class in her supper hour. "I'll give it a chance, and if it doesn't work, at least I can say I tried!"

Susan came to the first class with trepidation; she wasn't sure what to wear so had on jeans, a T-shirt and her black, lace-up prosthetic shoes. She told Sylvia later that night, "The Dojo is far too big-all that space that I have to cross doing this strange walk called 'half-mooning.' Worse, I have to return walking backwards! I just can't do it and I fall all the time and they make me get up and try it again!"

Susan tried wearing her sneakers at the next class, but with her lack of coordination coupled with her diabetic and MS peripheral neuropathy, she had no sensation of where her feet were on the floor, so again she stumbled and fell.

Determined to continue the classes, she wore her bedroom slippers next time, as she had always felt confident in walking around their old apartment with its slippery floors and many rugs with them on. Of course she received a lot of teasing but it was gentle and understanding, so she kept on going and learning. Before she could really believe it, she was moon-walking both forwards and backwards without a problem, as well as learning strikes, blocks, kenpos and combinations. She did fall-often-but she got up again and carried on.

Then six weeks into the class, she suffered a devastating stroke that left her unable to walk or move her arms and legs, puzzling her doctors because strokes are usually one-sided. She was in the hospital for a week and then in a rehabilitation facility where she was rapidly recovering when, three weeks after the first stroke she had an even more devastating event that left her totally deaf in one ear, unable to talk or to use her left side. After several more weeks in the hospital and in rehab, she came home, walking with a cane and unable to speak clearly or write.

Shawn, who had called or visited almost daily, insisted she came back to class. Sylvia juggled her schedule in order to drive Sue to the Dojo at least once a week, and she struggled through the classes with her quad cane for support, gradually improving and becoming more confident. Finally she was able to leave the cane by the wall.

Shawn suggested that it was time to give up the slippers and wear shoes more suitable for karate, and so she did, throwing the by now worn-out furry slippers into the back of her closet. Despite another stroke the next year, the worsening of her MS, Sylvia's retirement and their move to Belfast, Maine 110 miles north from the Dojo, she continued to go to classes, learn and advance in rank.

Now it is almost four years later. When she and Sylvia return home after she was awarded her green belt, she drags the slippers from the closet and nails them upon her Karate wall in their apartment, where all her certificates with their appropriate color belts are so proudly displayed.

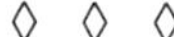

SYLVIA SIMS

When I do a form
I practice and practice
until I no longer
have to think about it.
I become that form.
I am that form.

My Chi is one with
every person
Who has become that form.

When I first accompanied Susan to the Dojo, little did I know that I would be standing by her almost four years later and receiving my green belt! After all, I was not physically disabled-unless you wanted to call being 68 years old with worn-out, arthritic knees disabled. I was still holding down a 32-hour week as an LPN in an extremely busy hospital unit as well as running a small business from my home as an editor, illustrator and book designer.

The first time I was able to accompany Sue, I sat down and prepared to relax and watch the class. There was quite a variety of students present, ranging from Sue in her white *gi* and belt through others with yellow and orange belts. Most of the students were visibly handicapped, some obviously from strokes, others from brain injuries and they varied in age from a couple of teenagers to several middle-aged and older men. Susan was the only female student, although there were two other women beside myself sitting in the back of the Dojo and watching. They introduced themselves as Sue and Peggy, wives and support persons to Linwood and Mo, both stroke victims.

Halfway through the class, Shawn urged the support people to join in. I was reluctant to make a fool of myself, but Peggy and Sue got up and I joined them, hanging in the back and attempting to learn half-mooning and some strikes. Before I knew it, I was swinging my arms and kiaing with enthusiasm. I was hooked!

Shawn explained to me after the class that Like Water had a policy of including support people in the monthly fee for the participant if they wanted to take the classes too, and he urged me to become the second woman in the class. So I bought a white gi and joined in whenever I was able to get a Wednesday or Friday evening off. When Sue returned to the class after her devastating strokes, she was no longer able to drive, so I scheduled my evening off on Fridays and attended regularly.

In fact I had been fascinated with martial arts for a long time; ever since I was sixteen years old and had been raped with ridiculous ease by a man not too much bigger than me, who held my arm behind my back in what he called a 'judo' hold and forced me face-down into the dirt. If I had attempted to struggle, I would have broken my arm. The pain and humiliation were terrible and I vowed to learn judo so that it would never happen again, but the opportunity was not there in impoverished, postwar Britain. I was a natural athlete; a dancer, a long-and high-jumper and a swimmer, so I did my best to learn jujitsu alone from a book from the library. College, marriage, motherhood, emigration, divorce, etcetera, intervened. When I moved to Portland, Maine in my '50s, my bank faced a Dojo on Congress Street and, trying not to be too obvious, I used to stare through the big windows at the students as I used the ATM, wishing I was younger. It did not occur to me that I was still in good shape, thanks to my habit of walking all over Portland plus my regular dance sessions at the local ballet studio, and could and should march over there and join in.

Here I am at 72 with two knee replacements that work splendidly. I have been studying with Like Water for four years, enjoying myself tremendously, getting to know two remarkable people-Shawn and Andrea-as well as a bunch of determined, equally remarkable men and women and now have a green belt that-believe me-I earned. I vow I will get my black belt even if it takes me until I am eighty!

Volunteer Teachers

NATHAN PROVENCHER, THE ZEN SENSEI

Nathan is fifteen years old, a second degree black belt and already an accomplished teacher. He has been volunteering with Like Water almost from the start. Students have seen him grow up and out of his childhood gi and almost out of his next one.

Nathan is a person of few words. When asked why he travels over 1 hour from Limington, Maine, to Scarborough to spend three hours of a Friday evening-precious to the average teenage boy-patiently teaching martial arts to students with many disabilities when he could be out with his friends, he replies, "I dunno. I just come . . . I like helping. It's something I do. It's here." When pressed, he admits that he likes martial arts and that he enjoys seeing "how much better the students are." He also appreciates the way that Andrea and Shawn include him in their trips to martial arts camps and to various conferences. Nathan has traveled with them to many local as well as out-of-state seminars.

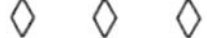

JULIE ENDRIZZI

Julie Endrizzi is a slender, dark, 16-year-old second degree black belt with an outgoing, enthusiastic personality. Both she and her younger brother, Doug, also a black belt as well as a champion swimmer, are volunteer instructors at Like Water.

"I have been studying karate all my life and love to teach. I love to see students do a form well and know that I taught them that. My father (an orthopedic surgeon) operated on Shawn's shoulder and told me about his program for the physically challenged, Like Water, and arranged an interview with him. Shawn was not in the least what I expected! He talked about his brain-injured students and told me I could do a lot for them. Shawn goes out of his way to help anyone who needs it and who has the will and the desire to respond. It is a fun learning experience and very gratifying.

"I want to go into medicine; probably surgery, maybe dermatology. I am taking an EMT course and this is a great learning experience for me, working with physically challenged people."

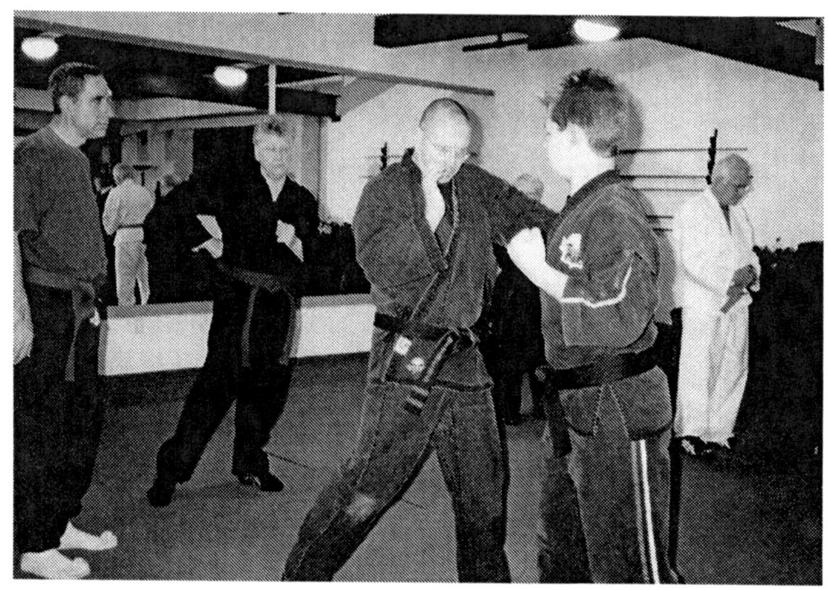

Teaching techniques with Nathan Provencher
(Also in photo: M. Schack, S. Sime, M. Tourigny)

Broken Wing Kenpo

A teacher affects eternity;
he can never tell where his influence stops.

Henry Brooks Adams,
from The Education of Henry Adams

As our school grows, we have come to realize that our experience and our students have had us make some significant changes in our curriculum-the one that we had studied-in order to make it challenging and beneficial to those students. We have worked on developing a unique and exciting style of martial arts that we have named Broken Wing Kenpo. Coming out of my frustration in adapting traditional martial arts to both my and my students' various abilities, it is based on traditional kenpo and designed specifically with the physically challenged in mind.

Broken Wing Kenpo is a style of martial arts based on kenpo and has been designed specifically with the physically challenged in mind. According to a Shaolin monk who was also a master of Kenpo, "Kenpo is the power of adaptability and yielding; the harmony of all things working together." It incorporates linear and circular movement to facilitate continuous motion, blending the dimensions of height, width, depth and time. It is based on logic: anticipating the moves of the opponent.

To this style we have included elements of Chi Kung, O-Ki-Tao and weapons-based styles as well as self-defense principles, blending the philosophy of Chinese, Japanese, Filipino and American martial arts. With Chi Kung, overall health is improved through combing the breath with certain gentle movements. The Japanese karate influence has an emphasis on concentrating as much of the body's power as possible at the point of impact, with timing, techniques and spirit considered as important as the physical. From the Chinese Kung Fu, comes the use of muscular coordination with a great awareness of the human skeletal and muscular anatomy and physiology as well as the fighting styles of animals. AMOK!, the system developed by Professor Tom Sotis, is based upon proven knife-fighting tactics of the

Filipino martial arts that can be adapted to any handheld object or to empty handed techniques. O-Ki-Tao-the Way of Ultimate Power developed by Douglas Young is a blend of practical street combat and martial arts.

This combination makes Broken Wing Kenpo a dynamic style that continually changes and grows with the student and the instructor. As with other styles of martial arts, it challenges and enhances the student's ability and provides a demanding workout. Practice of this art improves health and well-being by working the mind, body and spirit together. This style is well suited to

students with physical disabilities as well as those without. The versatility of Broken Wing Kenpo lies in the fact that it teaches effective skills to students with any degree of mobility- it lets the martial artist focus on their abilities, not their disabilities.

As this program is designed for students with physical disabilities, their safety and benefit are our highest priority, therefore the instructors alter and adapt each technique to each student's abilities. This curriculum is based on progressive principles with each subsequent skill building on the previous one. Rank is awarded based upon mastery of the appropriate levels of these principles.

Our teaching philosophy is that the knowledge of the martial arts is like building a house. The first part of the process is setting the foundation. It is plain concrete, but very strong. The next part is the shell of the house-the walls and the roof. These are also strong, but only as strong as the foundation they are set upon. The last part of the house is the décor and the trimming, and this is how we have set up the curriculum, in those three stages. In the beginning ranks we set the foundation. In the intermediate ranks, we build the shell of the house. In the advanced ranks, we put up the décor and smooth all the rough edges so that we ultimately end up with a strong masterpiece.

In order to advance to the next rank, tests are given. These periodic tests involve a review of techniques and abilities and, in order to provide a challenge for all students, short essays specific for their level may be required at the discretion of the chief instructor.

We also encourage our students to take an active role in their instruction and work with them to adapt their techniques to maximize their abilities. As students advance through the ranks they are encouraged to assist black belt instructors in teaching beginner's classes. It is our belief that teaching martial art makes us all better students of the arts.

Broken Wing Kenpo is a fluid style that will change with the growth of knowledge and the development of better techniques. Every student and teacher of the style will leave their fingerprints on its character.

This is only the beginning.

Afterword

When I started to study martial arts I was searching for something to further challenge myself both physically and mentally. I wanted to know how much I could take, how much I could really do. Ever since I was a kid I would always try to go beyond myself whether it was physical or mental. I was always testing my limits, not always safely, but I lived through it. Now I was older and the stroke had changed everything. It had woken me up, letting me know forcefully that it was time to get on the right track with my life. I had gotten back in shape by working out seven days a week so that I could get back to work. I got a great job, mastered it and then went on to college. When I was settled there, I needed more challenge.

As soon as I started martial arts, I realized that it was completely different from anything I had ever done. This was a group setting: I was used to working out alone. Being in a group, I was working at a far different and higher energy level than working out alone. It was a perfect challenge, even if there was a certain frustration in starting something new until I got in my groove. After a month or so, I noticed that, every time I got to a certain point, the energy level of the class was bumped up and I would have to move more quickly. I loved it. It kept me constantly challenged. As the weeks, months and tests went by, I noticed that I was stronger, quicker and was moving well. Mentally I was very alert and attentive. I realized quickly that I would never finish learning martial arts because there is so much to learn!

Reaching my black belt was just the beginning. I knew that I hadn't even scratched the surface of the wealth of knowledge available in martial arts, because you then move to a new level and start again. Every day is a new setting, a new challenge. It is never the same. I can play with everything I learn, adjust it and try a different way.

In teaching martial arts, I find that it is there for you as long as you want it to be. You can keep studying forever; there will always be something new to learn or a new way to do old techniques. I see things through my student's eyes and that keeps me energized and refreshed.

My philosophy has changed because I am constantly growing, sometimes in directions I had not anticipated. I know I will always come back to the basics, but on a different level. To me, martial arts is a continuing and growing lifetime journey if I allow it to be. I will always come back to the beginning, but with a little more experience each time and a different perspective as I constantly evolve. I have found this to be true in my teaching, too. Each day I may have the same class, but each day begins a new journey and a new adventure if I allow it to happen. Both Andrea and I want to do more. I have taught her the cane and she studies other styles as well, which is great as we share all our knowledge. I am truly the luckiest man alive to have such a dedicated wife and training partner who is my equal in every way and a far better martial artist. When she does form, she moves as if she is floating. She is extremely hard on herself and that makes her great.

It has been a little over ten years since I started

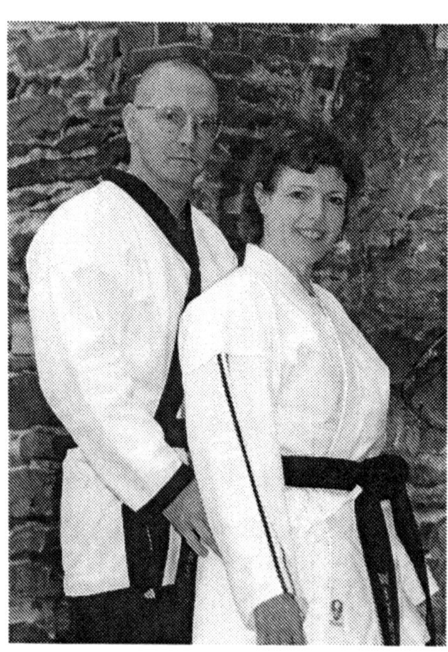

that journey. In the martial arts, that is not very much time. I am at the beginning again each day. I love it because every day I learn something new. I have grown immensely, but have never forgotten that first day. When I teach beginners, I try to be in their minds, to see martial arts from their perspective again and I learn new things.

I have made a choice: to continue to learn and grow and journey on the path.

Shawn Withers

DON'T QUIT

When things go wrong as they sometimes will,
When the road you're trudging seems all uphill,
When the funds are low and the debts are high,
And you want to smile, but you have to sigh,
When care is pressing you down a bit-
Rest if you must, but don't you quit.

Life is strange with its twists and turns,
As every one of us sometimes learns,
And many a person turns about
When they might have won if they stuck it out.

Don't give up though the pace seems slow-
You may succeed with another blow.
Often the struggler has given up
When he might have captured the victor's cup:
And he learned too late when the night came
down,
How close he was to the golden crown.

Success is failure turned inside out-
So stick to the fight when you're hardest hit-
It's when things seem the worst
That you mustn't quit!

Anonymous

Here is a Special Preview of Robert
Morgen's book

The Spiritually Aware Entrepreneur

A Step By Step Guide to Creating a
Simple and Affordable Business that
YOU Can Start
RIGHT NOW
(and use to make the world a better place!)

Introduction

We live in a very interesting time. There is an evolution in the business world and many of the conventional, accepted methods of earning a living are beginning to disappear. We've begun to move out of the Industrial Age and into the Information Age. Yet many of the attitudes and common teachings in our culture are still designed for success in the Industrial Age.

In many ways this is a very hard period for many people. We see the industrial jobs moving overseas and those cultures reaping the 'benefits' of industrialization, yet our schools, colleges and universities are still teaching people how to be successful employees in an industrial society.

This manual has been created as a resource for spiritually aware entrepreneurs who want to be self-employed while making the world a better place. It seems that many people who focus on their spirituality also believe that in order to be spiritual one must live in abject poverty.

I disagree.

In an infinite Universe there must exist both Infinite Abundance and Infinite Lack. This manual is about learning to tap into Infinite Abundance through personal development and financial education.

The Have's and Have Not's;

As the gap between the Have's and Have Not's continues to widen it's become apparent to me that one must make a conscious choice about which of these they want to be. I've noticed that we tend to create a paradox for ourselves when it comes to money and financial education. This paradox tends to spill over into every other part of our lives.

The Paradox;

We must be materially successful (to a certain point at least) in order to accomplish our goals. But in many people's opinion successful people (rich, wealthy, affluent, etc.) tend to have bad morals and be spiritually unhealthy.

This paradox creates a certain push-pull effect on our financial lives. For many people money still tends to be the deciding factor in almost every part of their lives. How often do we forego training and charitable opportunities because we feel that we "can't afford" to spend the money? How often would we like to do more to help with the various social issues that concern us, but feel that we are already at the limit of what we can *afford* to give? How many *good things* are NOT being accomplished because good people can't muster the resources to bring them to fruition?

A Radical Shift in Perspective

This manual will require a radical shift in perspective that many people simply won't be able to make. Those who've read my previous books will remember that I talk about making *incremental changes* in order to fully integrate the changes that we bring about in our lives. The principles that I write about here will hopefully help guide others into making those changes and creating an abundant and *sustainable* life.

The Spiritually Aware Entrepreneur

One of my long term goals is to begin creating a network of spiritually aware entrepreneurs. Some of you may have noticed that it's NOT the Politicians or "We the People" who run this country. It's the businesspeople!

Rather than complain about "the way things are", my goal is to create a network of people who are willing to put forth the effort and then put their money where their mouth is to create positive social and economic change. *It doesn't matter what religion or spiritual path you choose to pursue.* What matters is that you are interested in letting your heart, rather than your wallet, be your guide.

Starting and managing a business can be a great path for personal development and empowerment. It's a journey that will tax every resource that you can possibly muster, test your relationships, patience and resolve and teach you more than you probably wanted to know about yourself. It can also be one of the most fulfilling ways to spend your life, especially when you get to the point of being able to empower and support other people.

One of my goals with this book is to show that running a successful business is just as much a service as preaching to a congregation or administering to those who need physical or spiritual aid. Providing jobs, training and empowerment for people can be an important path to service and one that, when approached with the right attitude, can change the world.

The Tools

This book is more than just concepts and stories about the things that I screwed up on my journey. It also includes a comprehensive list of free tools and resources that you can begin using immediately to launch your new business. Using the tools and resources that I'll provide you'll be able to get products, create catalogs and blogs, set up marketing and advertising, sell your products and deposit the money in the bank and you'll be able to do all of that while sitting on the couch with your laptop.

All of the programs and software that you'll need will be included in the **Business in a Box** file that you'll be able to download for *free* from my website.

Terminology

This book is written for the preachers, clerics, healers, shamans, witches, witch doctors and other people who walk the spiritual pathways. It is meant to be completely non-denominational and it doesn't matter which religion, philosophy or deity that you subscribe to. In order to avoid all the clumsiness when referring to the various names, modalities and pathways I'm simply going to refer to us all as Lightworkers.

I've put a lot of jargon and technical terms in **bold**. Take some time and look these words up and do some web searches on them. I'm not going to put a Glossary in the back of the book because you'll learn far more by looking the words up online and then following the links you find than if I just told you what they mean.

Don't Take My Word For It!

I'm not going to use the word 'believe' or the phrase 'trust me' about any of the topics in this book. I want you to approach this book with a healthy dose of skepticism and give the tools and principles an honest try and see what happens. I'm writing about what has and hasn't worked for me and how I've pulled the various tools together. There are infinite variables here and this book should be taken as a general guide rather than as an instruction manual.

Software and Tools

Take your time when working with the tools and other software in the **Business in a Box** that accompanies this book. Don't buy any of the software programs until you've taken the time to learn to use the free versions that are included. I'm including the tools and software that I've found to be the best for what I'm doing. Most of these products were implemented after a stupidly long period of searching and experimenting. New products are always coming out and you may find that there are different products that suit your business.

Computer Skills

Face it; it's a digital world that we're moving into. To really implement the tools and software in the Business in a Box you should have a basic proficiency with the internet and computers.

Many of the programs use **PHP** and you'll need to be able to load them onto your server or web host and install them. This is actually a very simple process and the programs all have instructions in the **Readme** file. Be sure to take advantage of the Readme files and the **support forums** because the installation will vary depending upon your host.

DO NOT be intimidated by the software! I know some extremely technically deficient people who have been able to install and use these programs. You CAN do it, and the learning process will really open up your abilities with your business also.

Chapter 1
The Spiritually Aware Entrepreneur

The last couple of decades have seen an interesting evolution in the business world. Today we see people who create businesses in order to create positive change rather than going into business just to make money. We see people using the tools, cash flow and power that their business provides to create new jobs, fund charities and develop more resources and empowerment for the people around them.

Rather than embracing poverty and lack these entrepreneurs are opening themselves up to the unlimited abundance of the Universe and then using that abundance to help others. This is a major shift among those who walk a spiritual path. For a long time we've been trapped in the self-defeating paradigm that to be spiritual one must live in poverty and eschew all wealth and abundance.

Recent movies such as **The Secret** and **What the Bleep Do We Know?** have awakened millions of people to the **Law of Attraction** and the **Law of Reciprocity**. However this is NOT new information! *Napoleon Hill* published **Think and Grow Rich!** In the 1950's and *Wallace Wattles* published **The Science of Getting Rich** in 1910! **The Science of Getting Rich** was one of the books used as the basis for **The Secret**.

So what has changed recently to cause this shift in awareness about abundance? The information has always been there. The simple fact is that many spiritually oriented people saw wealth as evil or bad. I can't tell you how many times I've met Lightworkers who held full-time jobs and then spent their 'spare time' teaching and healing, often for free. In almost every case, when asked about money the Lightworker would respond "Money isn't important to me." Well, if money is not important then why are we spending 40-60 hours a week working for it and then teaching and healing on the side? If our true path is to be teachers, healers and Lightworkers then shouldn't we be doing that rather than working a job that we probably don't like in order to pay the bills?

I don't want it to seem as if I'm criticizing these people who work so hard to help others. That's not my intention at all. I simply want to point out that those folks could be helping so many *more* people if they didn't have to spend so much time working for something (money) that they don't think is important in the first place!

The last few years have seen a major attitude shift as these same Lightworkers have started to see that it's OK to be paid for their time, skill and education. Why shouldn't it be? Some Western doctors have charged exorbitant fees for decades on the premise that they should be reimbursed for the years of college and the expenses incurred there. The average Lightworker probably has at least as much education and training as the average medical doctor. I know people who have studied and trained for *decades* in order to be able to teach and heal for free! The insanity of this double standard never ceases to amaze me and I'm thrilled to see us finally beginning to move beyond it.

Money as a Tool

Today more and more spiritually oriented people are beginning to view money as a tool that can help them to be more effective in their life's work. To these people having a lot of money is not about a big house or a fancy car or any of the ego bound trappings of wealth. Rather it's about being able to promote their classes and create better materials and tools for their students and being able to empower more people.

The reality of our modern world is that money *is* important. Very few of us are willing to give away everything we own and live a path of poverty and asceticism as an example to others. While I'm certainly not knocking that path and those called to it, the point here is that there are other paths and other groups of people that we have to make contact with.

The ability to use money effectively and manifest abundance is a skill set of its own. It's what the rest of this book is about.

Chapter 2
Where We Came From and Where We're Going

Many Lightworkers today are still working under the tribal attitudes that probably carry over from past lives when we were shamans, healers and tribal medicine men. In those days and places we didn't have to fool with 'making a living', we could just live and take care of the tribe and the tribe took care of us.

Now the world has evolved and there are new ways and new attitudes. We still need to take care of the tribe and the tribe is happy to take care of us, but all too often it's *we Lightworkers* who aren't making the shift into this new world and it's actually causing problems for the tribe.

We're seeing an interesting revival of the Old Ways now. Some of the modern religions have done a good job of providing a framework for laws and social norms and mores, not to mention fodder for countless wars and atrocities, but it seems that they've left a lot of people looking for spirituality rather than providing an easy path to help integrate the body, mind and spirit and many people are actively beginning to seek alternative paths. These are our tribe; the seekers, the wanderers and those open-minded souls who intuitively feel that they should be looking inside themselves for the divinity that they can sense rather than looking outward to the invisible Gods that are forced upon them.

A Lightworker is always going to be in the position of straddling the boundaries between the various realities. We don't believe in the Universal Powers and the Universal Laws, we *know* that they are real and that they work because we've felt and experienced them.

One of our missions is to help awaken others to those powers, and in many cases those others don't believe that the powers actually exist because they have been taught that they have to be able to scientifically prove their concepts before they can be free to believe in them.

At the same time the people that we are supposed to be helping to awaken are indoctrinated from birth into mainstream religions that tell them to have faith in the religious version of the supernatural while teaching that all other versions of the supernatural are unreal and evil. It's no wonder that the tribe is confused and looking for relief and answers.

Another problem here is that many of the Lightworkers are still breaking free of the attitudes and teachings of the mainstream religions. It's hard to grow up being taught that "money is the root of all evil" and then being put into a position where one must learn to use money as a tool in order to help the tribe. Many Lightworkers feel that to accept money for teaching or healing actually sullies the teaching and healing and lessens its worth. I've also met Lightworkers who have difficulties *accepting* money or even bartered goods that are offered in exchange for teaching and healing.

The tribe, on the other hand, is being taught that *"you get what you pay for"* because they are being indoctrinated into a consumer oriented society. When a Lightworker offers a service then the tribe expects to pay for that service just as they would pay a doctor or a plumber or a school teacher. When a Lightworker has an inner conflict over accepting payment it actually *interrupts the flow of energy* that exists between the tribe and the Lightworkers! We can't teach that "energy doesn't flow through tight muscles" and then create *resistance* to our energy flows.

In the times before the industrial revolution and the rise of the consumer oriented cultures Light workers only had to straddle 2 worlds. We had to keep one foot out in the Universe and the other foot here in the collective illusion that the tribe creates as it flows along its daily path to awakening.

Today we have to straddle 3 worlds. The Universe and the illusion are still there and we have to help bridge the gap between these for the tribe, but we also have to stay tapped into the financial world created by the consumerism of the modern times. The problem for many of us is that we literally don't have a leg to stand on when it comes to this new consumer society and no one has ever taught us how to integrate it into our teachings and practices in any useful way. In fact we've been taught that consumerism is bad and we've believed it *even while espousing balance and harmony*! We can just add this to the growing list of inner conflicts that are blocking our energy. I hope the tools and exercises in the book are helpful with balancing out some of those conflicts.

Consumerism and the modern world

Sometimes it can be hard to balance the realities of the worlds we straddle. We can directly attribute much of the rise of the New Age to the books and media distributed throughout our consumer society. In fact the tools and technologies of the Information Age have made it easier than ever before to develop a healing and teaching practice. There has never been a time in the known history of the human race when the common people, the regular, ordinary working people, have had access to the writings and teachings of every great discipline that has survived the purges of the religions and ravages of time.

Today we can go to the bookstore, visit the library and read the websites and find vast amounts of information and guidance that previously would have been available only to the priests and royalty. Lightworkers have the ability to teach, heal and reach across vast distances to help the members of their tribe.

Today the members of our tribes are scattered and it's up to each of us to find them and then help provide the healing, teaching and guidance that they might need. We may not always be able to meet them face to face or heal them directly as in the old days, but that simply means that the modern Lightworker has to be more versatile, persistent and tolerant than ever before.

Chapter 3
The Global Economy

Hardly a day goes by when the news channels don't tell of how another business has outsourced its labor force to a 3rd World country. It's a process that has devastated American communities and created a vast amount of ill will and bad feelings toward the businesses that have done the outsourcing. It's also creating a gulf between American consumers and those who actually make the products now.

The real problem here is not the jobs that are exported or the products that are imported, but the attitudes and ideas that have been indoctrinated into us along the way.

As recently as a hundred years ago most Americans made a certain amount of their income independently, rather than working for it in a factory. Over 95% of the people grew some portion of their own food and many of these took their excess to be sold in the various markets that existed then. They also made a wide variety of other products, crafts and forms of art which they also sold and bartered.

The Industrial Revolution changed all that. In an eye blink we discovered that most of us now had jobs in factories and that we were drawing a paycheck rather than having to work in the fields and make products to be sold independently. In the beginning this was a refreshing change because the entrepreneur's lifestyle that we formerly lived was fraught with insecurity and instability. Now we could put a dollar value on our time and know exactly how much money we'd be bringing home on payday.

Of course the trade off was that we didn't have time to make many of the products that we used to create for our daily use, but that was a minor problem and we could use the cash flow from the industrial job to just buy those items that we used to make or trade for.

For awhile the prosperity of the Industrial Age made it easy to ignore the fact that we were trading our freedoms for our new notions of security. The advancements in technology brought new vaccines and medicines as well as new media technologies. We even changed our school systems because we needed to create more literate employees and workers.

It's only when the industrial jobs go away that we realize that we no longer have the skills or attitudes to survive independently. Now all of our food is brought in from other parts of the country or the world and we don't know how to grow our own even if we wanted to.

We also find ourselves trapped by the same consumerism that we embraced so readily decades ago. We don't have the skills or even the raw materials to create the tools and items that we need on a daily basis nor do the markets still exist where we can easily barter and trade for them.

So here we stand, cast aside by the great machine and without the skills, abilities and resources to live and survive in the way we've been taught. At the same time we see others embracing the industrial jobs that were once ours, and embracing the same attitudes and affluence.

But is the situation really that bleak?

While this can be a confusing time for many people we should also remember that the only real constant is change! We've left the Industrial Age behind and we stand on the threshold of the Information Age.

Attitudes and Opportunity

"When you ask for patience God doesn't give you patience, He gives you opportunities to be patient. If you ask for courage He doesn't just give you courage, He gives you opportunities to be courageous."
Morgan Freeman (as God) in *Evan Almighty*

The average American has never been as readily poised to take advantage of an evolving situation as we are right now. The proliferation of the internet and the availability of computers has put us in a position where we can almost instantly start going back to our entrepreneurial roots. America wasn't built by factory workers longing for security and steady jobs, it was hacked out of the wilderness and stolen from the natives by people who wanted to live free and have the ability to prosper based upon their own merits and willingness to work hard!

There were no glass ceilings when we started building this country. Hey, we barely even had roofs. People didn't complain that the government didn't take care of them, they came here *to get away from* governments that wouldn't let them breathe freely and grow, governments that taxed them (for their own good) and regulated them (for their own good) and restricted them.

Our forefathers established new frontiers and created new products and then created markets for those products. Today we have different frontiers and new and different products and the ability to create new and wondrous markets not for greed and avarice, but to help and empower others.

Today we have the ability to start gathering our tribes and healing the planet in ways that we never could have imagined before. The new frontiers are within and around us as we rediscover our cosmic connections and the oneness of the abundant Universe that we're all a part of. We have a growing tribe that needs our help to learn how to reconnect to energies from which we've been estranged for hundreds of years. That tribe is scattered all over the world and rather than being divided by oceans and mountains we're finding ourselves connected by industry and commerce.

It's going to take some radical shifts in attitude, but we have the technology and the information to make that shift ourselves and then demonstrate the shift to others and *we don't even have to work at it full-time*!

We can use **leverage** and **passive marketing** to create new **income streams** to help those who are disadvantaged financially. We can create products that increase the awareness of the abundance of the Universe and help our tribe begin to once again connect to its unlimited potential. We can use the internet, audio, video and print media to create new markets that span the globe and create new jobs while empowering those around us in ways that our parent's generation couldn't even imagine. We can use the *passive income* from our new media and methodologies to support the charities and social programs that we believe in and literally begin changing the world!

So with that said, let's get started!

Books and CDs from Mystic Wolf Press

Item	Price	S&H
Kundalini Awakening for Personal Mastery 2nd Edition	$16.95	$3.00
Easy Meditation for Martial Artists	$16.95	$3.00
Easy Meditation CD Set (Includes all 4 CDs)	$74.95	$5.00
Easy Introduction to Meditation CD	$19.95	$3.00
Advanced Meditation Exercises CD	$19.95	$3.00
Timed Meditation Music Tracks CD	$19.95	$3.00
Opening the Chakras CD	$29.95	$3.00
The Spiritually Aware Entrepreneur	$16.95	$3.00
Broken Wing	$16.95	$3.00
Total		

Special Offer!

Free shipping on all orders over $100.
ALL of Robert Morgen's books come signed by the author. Please let us know if you'd like a special inscription in your copy.

Please make your check or money order out to
Mystic Wolf Press, Inc.

Send your order to :
Mystic Wolf Press
11661 W. 14th Ave
Golden, CO 80401

Watch our website for more products coming soon. For samples of the CDs visit the 'Kundalini Awakening with Robert Morgen' Podcast.

www.mysticwolfpress.com

Printed in the United States
200557BV00002B/1-105/A